PROSTATE CANCER C
FOR SENIORS

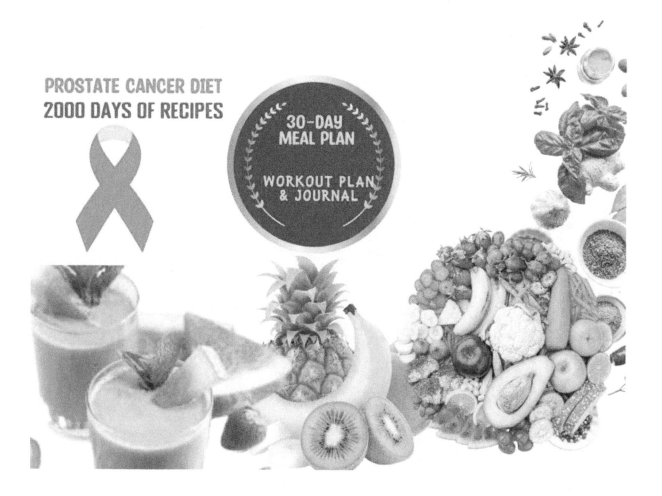

PROSTATE CANCER DIET
2000 DAYS OF RECIPES

30-DAY
MEAL PLAN

WORKOUT PLAN
& JOURNAL

Comprehensive Nourishing Recipes for Cancer
Recovery with Meal Plans to Support Healthy Living

Dr. Gerry D. Reyna

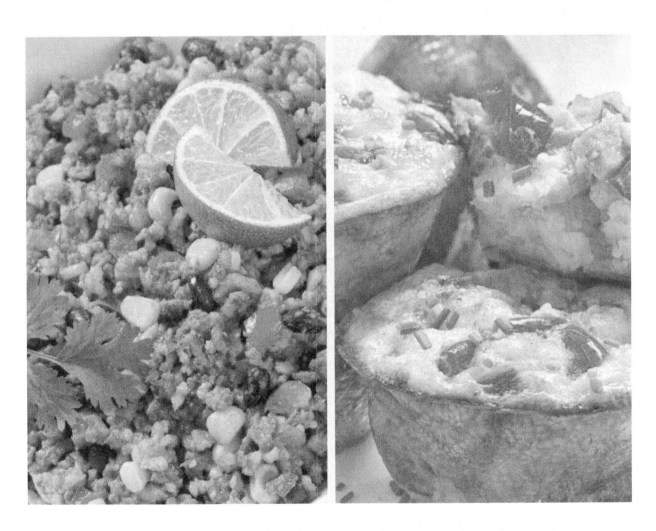

TABLE OF CONTENTS

1. Read the Introduction: Start by reading the introduction to the cookbook. This section usually provides background information on prostate cancer, diet guidance, and the overall purpose of the book.

2. Review the Nutritional Information: Look for sections that outline the nutritional benefits of specific ingredients or recipes. Pay special attention to guidance for key nutrients that are important for prostate cancer patients, such as antioxidants, fiber, and healthy fats.

3. Check for Meal Plans: Some cookbooks may include sample meal plans for seniors with prostate cancer. Analyze these plans to understand how to structure your meals for optimal nutrition and health benefits.

4. Assess the Recipes: Take a closer look at the recipes provided in the cookbook. Consider the ingredients used, cooking methods, portion sizes, and nutritional content. Look for recipes that include a variety of nutrient-dense foods and focus on anti-inflammatory and immune-boosting ingredients.

5. Consider Personal Preferences and Diet Restrictions: Keep in mind your personal preferences, diet restrictions, and any specific guidance from your healthcare provider. Choose recipes that align with your tastes and diet needs while still supporting your prostate cancer treatment.

6. Plan Your Meals: Use the cookbook to plan your meals for the week ahead. Select a variety of recipes that offer a balance of nutrients and flavors. Make a shopping list based on the ingredients needed for the recipes you've chosen or follow the example inside the book.

7. Prepare and Cook: Follow the instructions provided in the cookbook to prepare and cook the recipes. Take your time in the kitchen, enjoy the process of cooking, and enjoy the delicious and nutritious meals you've created.

8. Monitor Your Health: As you implement recipes from the cookbook into your diet, pay attention to how you feel physically and emotionally. Monitor any changes in your symptoms, energy levels, digestion, and overall well-being

YOU'RE NOT ALONE!

The health of the prostate is crucial for men, given that it is a gland responsible for producing fluid for semen and assisting in urine regulation. The prostate can be impacted by three primary conditions: prostatitis, benign prostatic hyperplasia, and prostate cancer. In order to mitigate or lower the risk of these conditions, it is recommended that men sustain a healthy weight, increase their intake of vegetables, limit the consumption of red meat, and undergo regular testing.

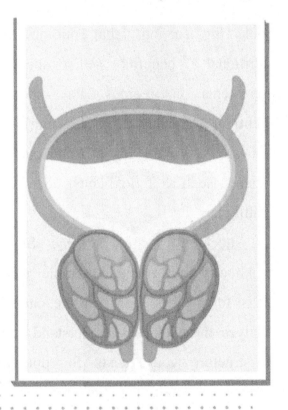

INTRODUCTION TO PROSTATE CANCER COOKBOOK FOR SENIORS

Prostate Cancer Cookbook for Seniors is a comprehensive guide designed to support the health and well-being of older adults dealing with prostate cancer. This cookbook provides practical and accessible resources to help seniors improve their process with prostate cancer through the power of nutrition and healthy eating.

Meet Graham, a 75-year-old man who was diagnosed with prostate cancer. The news was a shock, but Graham decided to fight back with the help of food. He started using the "**Prostate Cancer Cookbook for Seniors**" to transform his diet and his life.

Graham began including more fruits and vegetables in his meals, focusing on foods known to promote prostate health. He experimented with new recipes, from hearty soups filled with cancer-fighting ingredients to colorful salads bursting with nutrients. With each bite, Graham felt satisfied, knowing that he was taking control of his health.

Over time, Graham's dedication to his new diet paid off. His energy levels improved, and he felt stronger. His regular check-ups showed promising results, and most importantly, Graham felt a renewed sense of hope and optimism for the future.

One afternoon, as Graham enjoyed a meal of grilled salmon with a side of roasted vegetables, he reflected on his journey. He had not only survived prostate cancer but had thrived in old age. Through the power of food and determination, Graham had reversed the course of his illness and emerged stronger.

As we age, our bodies undergo changes that can increase the risk of developing prostate cancer. However, research has shown that certain dietary choices and lifestyle habits can play a crucial role in managing this condition and improving the overall quality of life. By making informed decisions about the foods we eat, seniors can take control of their health and well-being in the face of prostate cancer.

In this cookbook, you will find a wealth of delicious and nutritious recipes specifically adjusted to meet the unique nutritional needs of seniors with prostate cancer. Each recipe has been carefully created to include ingredients that are known to promote prostate health and support the body's natural defenses against cancer. From hearty soups and salads to satisfying main dishes and delectable desserts, these recipes are designed to be simple, easy to prepare, and most importantly, enjoyable to eat.

Whether you are a senior facing a recent diagnosis of prostate cancer or a caregiver looking to support a loved one through their journey, this cookbook is your go-to resource for nourishing meals that prioritize health and well-being. By accepting the power of food as medicine and making positive changes to your diet, you can take proactive steps towards managing prostate cancer and living a healthier, more fulfilling life.

Key Benefits Of A Prostate Cancer Diet For Seniors

1. Improved Prostate Health: The diet is rich in nutrients and antioxidants that support prostate health. This can potentially reduce inflammation, support immune function and promote overall prostate wellness.

2. Cancer-Fighting Properties: The diet includes many foods connected to anti-cancer properties. A diet rich in fruits, vegetables, whole grains, and lean proteins may help the body fight off cancer cells and reduce the risk of cancer recurrence.

3. Reduced Inflammation: The diet is rich in anti-inflammatory foods such as fruits, vegetables, whole grains, and healthy fats. This can help reduce inflammation in the body, which is important for managing cancer and supporting overall health.

4. Supports Immune Function: The nutrient-dense foods in the diet can boost the immune system. This helps seniors fight off infections and illnesses while undergoing cancer treatment.

5. Promotes Heart Health: Many components of the diet, such as omega-3 fatty acids from fish, fiber from whole grains, and antioxidants from fruits and vegetables, can also benefit heart health and reduce the risk of cardiovascular diseases.

6. Enhanced Digestive Health: A diet high in fiber and hydration can support digestive health, prevent constipation, and promote regular bowel movements. This is important for seniors undergoing cancer treatment.

7. Maintains Muscle Mass: Adequate protein intake from sources like lean meats, poultry, fish, and plant-based proteins can help seniors maintain muscle mass and strength. This is crucial for overall health and quality of life.

8. Balanced Blood Sugar Levels: Choosing whole, unprocessed foods in the diet can help regulate blood sugar levels. This reduces the risk of diabetes and promotes stable energy levels throughout the day.

9. Improved Mental Health: Eating a nutrient-rich diet can also have positive effects on mental health. It promotes cognitive function, mood stability, and overall well-being during the challenges of prostate cancer treatment.

10. Supports Bone Health: Including foods rich in calcium, vitamin D, and other nutrients essential for bone health can help seniors maintain strong bones and reduce the risk of osteoporosis. This may be particularly important during cancer treatment.

11. Weight Management: Following a prostate cancer diet that focuses on whole, unprocessed foods can help seniors maintain a healthy weight. Excess weight has been linked to an increased risk of cancer and other chronic diseases, so maintaining a healthy weight through a diet can be crucial for overall health.

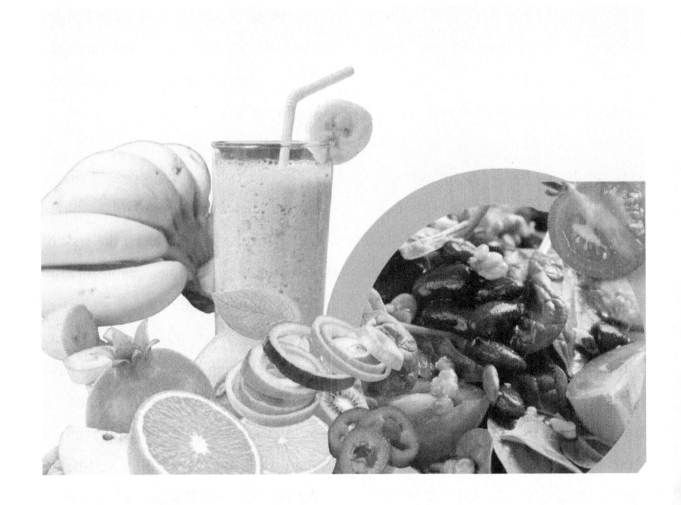

CHAPTER 1: PROSTATE CANCER IN ADULTS

Prostate cancer is a common health concern among older men, with the median age of diagnosis being 66 years. A significant proportion of patients, 60%, are diagnosed when they are over 65 years old, and 20% are diagnosed when they are over 75 years old. Despite the high incidence of prostate cancer in older men, it's unclear whether older men benefit from the same treatment strategies used in younger men. This is because older patients and those with more health conditions are often underrepresented in clinical trials.

Older patients usually have more health conditions and less physical functional reserve, which is the difference between a person's maximum physical capacity and the minimum necessary to perform daily functions. Therefore, they may benefit from treatment approaches that are peculiar to their specific needs and circumstances.

The first step in developing a tailored approach is to assess a patient's overall health status. This includes a frailty assessment to align treatment recommendations with each patient's goals and ability to tolerate treatment. Weakness is a state of vulnerability to external stressors, leading to poor health outcomes. Frail patients experience declines in multiple physiological systems, resulting in decreased mobility, muscle strength, bone density, balance, motor processing, cognition, endurance, and physical activity.

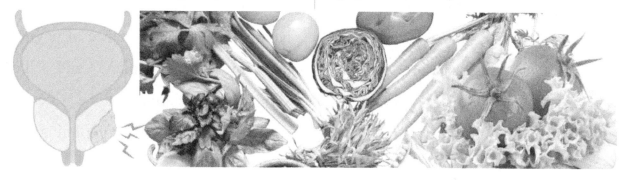

The biology of frailty is complex, involving inflammation, loss of stem-cell regeneration, DNA damage, metabolic decline, hormone dysregulation, epigenetic changes, and loss of proteostasis. More than half of older patients with cancer are estimated to have either prefrailty or weakness. One significant contributor to frailty is a decrease in testosterone. It's estimated that 50%-80% of men older than 80 years have hypogonadism, which is associated with decreased muscle mass and bone density, as well as increased falls.

This is particularly relevant to men with prostate cancer because the treatment of advanced and metastatic disease relies on androgen deprivation therapy (ADT), which depletes testosterone and can accelerate weakness. In one group of prostate cancer survivors, those who had current or previous exposure to ADT were more than twice as likely to be classified as prefrail or frail (40%-43%) compared with those never exposed to ADT (15%). Even short courses of ADT can result in sarcopenia, muscle weakness, declines in bone mineral density (BMD), fatigue, reduced activity levels, and falls.

Identifying frailty or prefrailty in men with prostate cancer can guide the Health Center in deciding whether to offer prostate cancer-directed treatment and in identifying interventions that improve the patient's physical reserve. The first part of this discussion focuses on risk assessment and decision-making tools that can be used in managing older men with prostate cancer. Along with implementing these assessment tools in the expert health center, it's crucial to have a plan for addressing the potential deficits identified. Studies have shown the importance of having an intervention plan and the significant variation in the rate of interventions after completing a geriatric assessment (GA).

The second part of this discussion will focus on specific interventions that can reduce weakness and improve treatment tolerance in men with prostate cancer, highlighting evidence from prospective studies of interventions that may comprehensively address weakness among men with prostate cancer. The final section will discuss how to integrate the use of assessment tools and interventions with recent treatment advances in prostate cancer while also considering the social determinants of health for each individual.

Prostate cancer, excluding skin cancer, is the most common type of cancer in men in the U.S. In 2022, the American Cancer Society estimated that nearly 270,000 men would be diagnosed with prostate cancer. The average age of diagnosis is 66, and as men age, their chances of developing the disease increase. The most predominant questions of whether to screen for prostate cancer and whether to treat it become more complex with age. However, the disease can be more deadly for older individuals. According to guidelines from the American Society of Cancer Health Center, prostate cancer is more than twice as likely in people over 70 than in younger people. They're also more than 4 times as likely to have advanced prostate cancer and are more likely to die from the disease.

However, it's important to remember that age is just a number. While the risk increases with each day, there's no specific age at which prostate cancer becomes most dangerous. When discussing diagnosis and treatment options with your experts, the focus should not only be on your chronological age—the number of years you've been alive—but also on your biological age as well.

Biological age refers to your current health status based on factors like your genes, lifestyle, and environment. Are you fit and otherwise healthy? Or do you have other illnesses that affect your overall health? This can help predict a healthy lifespan.

For instance, two men who are both 70 years old have the same chronological age. But if one of them has been a lifelong smoker, his biological age is probably higher. He has an increased risk of dying from smoking-related health problems like heart disease and lung disease. A man with a lower biological age may be more likely to benefit from prostate cancer treatment. Guidelines advise offering treatment only to those who are expected to live 10 or more years, regardless of their age. If they are, treatment decisions are the same as for younger people.

How Does Treatment Differ When You Are Adult?

As individuals age, the likelihood of developing chronic diseases such as heart disease and diabetes increases. This can complicate treatment decisions. For instance, hormone deprivation treatment, also known as androgen suppression treatment, is often used to slow the progression of prostate cancer. While it's not a cure, it can help manage the disease for some time.

However, there are concerns associated with hormone deprivation treatment. Some research, though not all, suggests that it may increase the risk of high blood pressure, diabetes, heart disease, and stroke. It might even increase the likelihood of dying from heart disease. Other potential side effects of hormone deprivation treatment include weakened bones, leading to a condition called osteoporosis, and an increased risk of fractures. It can also lead to cognitive issues.

Therefore, the risks of treatment need to be weighed against its potential benefits by medical doctors.

A study conducted in 2008 examined over 200,000 men with prostate cancer aged between 65 and 84. The researchers found that only those with the most advanced cases of prostate cancer were more likely to die from their cancer than from another cause. Interestingly, men in the study had a much higher chance of dying from heart failure than from late-stage prostate cancer. This highlights the importance of considering overall health and other potential risks when making treatment decisions for prostate cancer.

Alternative Treatments Will Reduce The Symptoms And Side Effects Of Prostate Cancer

1. **Lycopene:** Some fruits and vegetables, particularly stewed tomatoes, contain high levels of this potent antioxidant. Some research shows that diets heavy on tomatoes and other lycopene-rich foods reduce cancer risk.

2. **Pomegranate Juice:** In mouse experiments, pomegranate has been proven to reduce the growth of cancer cells. Research on human cells shows similar capacity.

3. **Green Tea:** Some research studies indicate that green tea may have cancer-fighting effects.

4. **Shiitake Mushroom Extract:** Shiitake mushrooms are thought to have immune-boosting and anti-cancer properties.

5. **Modified Citrus Pectin (MCP):** MCP is a fiber generated from citrus fruits that is considered to have anti-cancer properties.

6. **Mind-Body Practices:** Yoga, meditation, and massage can help reduce the adverse effects of therapy and the stress of a cancer diagnosis.

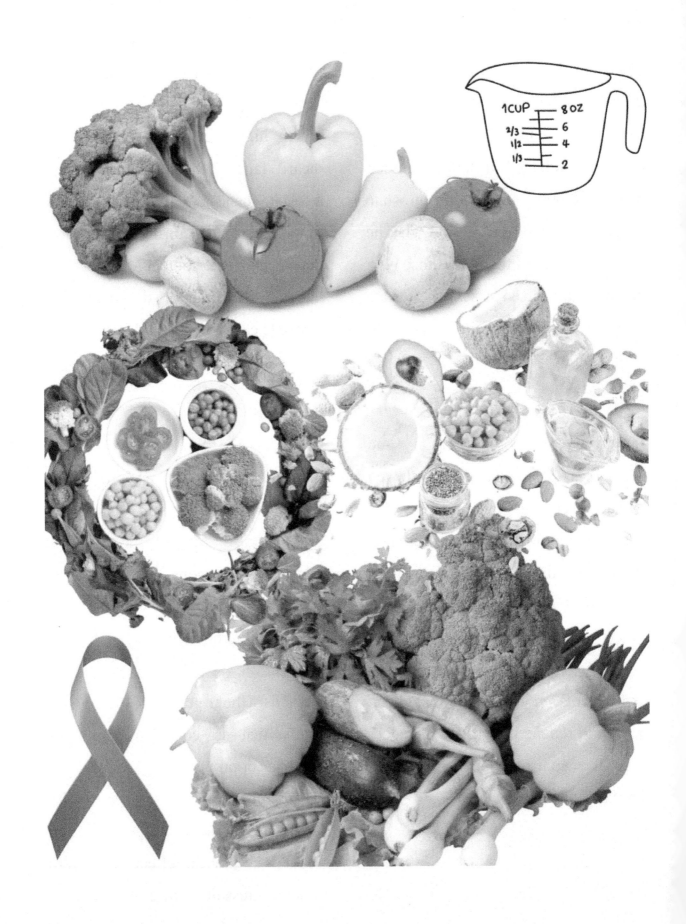

CHAPTER 2: GROCERY SHOPPING LIST

FRUITS AND VEGETABLES

Berries (fresh or frozen)
Bok choy
Broccoli
Brussels sprouts
Cauliflower
Edamame
Garlic
Grapes
Grapefruits
Leafy greens (such as spinach and romaine lettuce)
Oranges
Pears
Sweet potatoes
Tomatoes
Bell Peppers
Carrots
Kiwi
Avocado
Red Cabbage
Zucchini
Green Beans
Cranberries

PROTEINS

Fish (Rich In Omega-3 Fatty Acids)
Lean Chicken Or Turkey
Tofu
Black, Red, Or Pinto Beans
Garbanzo Beans (Chickpeas)
Lentils
Eggs Or Egg Substitutes
Mushroom
Kidney Beans
Tuna
Salmon
Cod
Sea Food
Edamame
Tempeh
Chickpeas (Garbanzo Beans)
Almonds
Walnuts
Pistachios

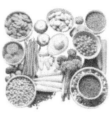

BEVERAGES

Green or white tea
Water
Coffee

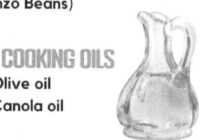

COOKING OILS

Olive oil
Canola oil

HERBS AND SPICES

Cumin (Jeera)
Fennel (Saunf
Mint (Pudina)
Turmeric
Ginger
Rosemary

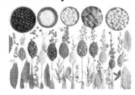

DAIRY

Skim milk
Low-fat cheese
Rice milk
Almond milk
Hemp milk
Soy milk
Coconut milk
Cashew milk
Dairy alternatives (such as soy-based foods and nut milk)

WHOLE GRAINS

Barley
Buckwheat
Millet
Spelt
Wild rice or brown rice
Whole grain pasta
Whole grain bread, tortillas, or buns
Oatmeal
Quinoa

Foods Can Worsen Prostate Cancer

1. Non-Grass-Fed Beef: Beef that is produced on a large scale and fed with substances such as corn, grain, and soy can trigger chemical reactions in the bovine digestive system. There is a 12% higher risk of prostate cancer in men who consume beef that is not grass-fed, compared to those who opt for organic, grass-fed beef.

2. Non-Organic Chicken: Chickens that are raised in industrial farming environments frequently receive hormones, antibiotics, and steroids. These chickens have been found to contain heterocyclic amines. Studies have demonstrated that these compounds can cause prostate cancer in rats and inflict DNA damage in human prostate tissue grown in a lab.

3. Dairy: The saturated fats in most dairy products can undermine the overall low-fat diet that is best for prostate health. It's better to get your calcium from salmon, greens, and almonds instead of dairy.

4. Caffeine: Caffeine functions as a diuretic, which can intensify the need to urinate. This could pose difficulties for individuals with an enlarged prostate, leading to discomfort.

5. Spicy And Acidic Foods: The consumption of these foods can lead inflammation in the bladder and prostate, which can exacerbate the primary urinary symptoms in men who are dealing with compromised prostate health.

6. Alcohol: The consumption of alcohol can heighten the need to urinate, which may result in irritation of both the bladder and the prostate.

7. Sweet Baked Goods: Foods that are high in saturated fats can potentially exacerbate the symptoms associated with prostate disease.

8. Some Salad Dressings: A significant number of salad dressings use saturated fats to achieve their desired consistency. These fats can adhere to the salad and may potentially hurt prostate health.

9. Saturated Fats In Any Food: Saturated fats have been linked to heart disease, and recent studies indicate a potential association between the intake of saturated fats and an increased risk of prostate cancer.

10. Excess Calcium: While calcium is beneficial for health, an overconsumption of calcium has been linked to the proliferation of tumor tissue in individuals who are already diagnosed with prostate cancer

CHAPTER 3: BREAKFAST RECIPES FOR PROSTATE CANCER

1. Quinoa Breakfast Bowl With Berries And Almond

Quinoa is a protein-rich grain that serves as a solid basis for a variety of toppings. When mixed with berries and almonds, it creates a meal that is not only delicious but also high in antioxidants and essential nutrients.

INGREDIENTS

- 1 cup of quinoa (rinsed)
- 2 cups of almond milk (or any other milk of your choice)
- 1/2 teaspoon of ground cinnamon
- 1 tablespoon of maple syrup (you can adjust to taste)
- 1/2 cup of fresh berries (strawberries, blueberries, or raspberries)
- 1/4 cup of almonds (sliced)

INSTRUCTIONS

1. In a medium saucepan, mix the rinsed quinoa and almond milk. Stir in the cinnamon.

2. Bring the mixture to a boil and then lower it to a simmer. Place the cover on and cook for 15-20 minutes, until the quinoa has absorbed most of the milk.

3. Remove from the heat and add the maple syrup.

4. Serve the quinoa in bowls and top it with fresh berries and sliced almonds.

COOKING TIPS

1. Before adding the milk, roast the quinoa in the pot for a few minutes to improve its flavor.

2. Prepare the quinoa ahead of time and reheat it in the morning for a quick breakfast.

Nutritional Values Per Serving: Calories: Approximately 279 | Carbohydrates: 55g | Fat: 4g | Protein: 8g

SERVING PORTION: THIS RECIPE SERVES 2.

PREP TIME: 5 MINUTES

COOK TIME: 20 MINUTES

NOTE

1. Cooked broccoli or cauliflower can be served on the side.

2. Add a few slices of cooked tomatoes, which are high in lycopene.

3. Quinoa and almonds are high in protein and healthy fats.

4. Almond milk makes an excellent alternative to full milk.

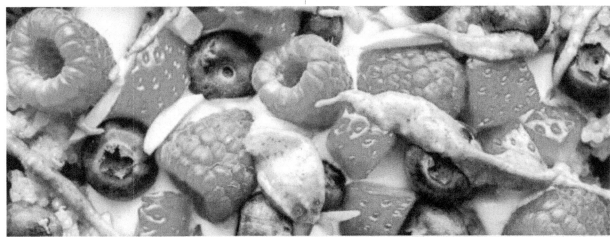

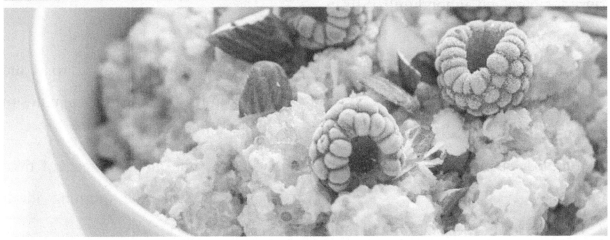

2. Vegetable And Tofu Scramble

This Vegetable and Tofu Scramble is an important and nutritious meal, perfect for seniors on a prostate cancer diet. It includes plant-based proteins and a variety of veggies, making it an ideal way to start the day.

INGREDIENTS

- 1 ½ teaspoons of extra-virgin olive oil
- 5 ounces of extra-firm tofu, drained and cubed
- 1 cup of chopped vegetables (such as zucchini, mushrooms, and onions)
- 1/2 teaspoon of spice of choice (e.g., chili powder or ground cumin)
- Pinch of ground pepper
- 1/3 cup of canned chickpeas, rinsed
- 1/4 cup of pico de gallo or salsa
- 1/4 cup of shredded Cheddar cheese, preferably sharp (1 oz.)

INSTRUCTIONS

1. Heat the olive oil in a large, nonstick pan over medium-high heat.

2. Add the tofu, vegetables, chosen spice, and pepper; cook, stirring often, until the vegetables are softened, about 5 to 7 minutes.

3. Add the chickpeas and pico de gallo (or salsa) and cook for 1 to 2 minutes.

4. Remove from heat, arrange the scramble into one corner of the pan, cover with Cheddar cheese, and let it melt.

5. If preferred, add more spicy sauce and chopped cilantro.

COOKING TIPS

1. Feel free to make this scramble using your favorite vegetables.

2. For the best results, cook veggies at the same rate.

Nutritional Values Per Serving: Calories: Approximately 420 | Fat: 26g | Carbohydrates: 26g | Protein: 27g

SERVING PORTION: THIS RECIPE YIELDS 2 3/4 CUPS, SERVING 1.

PREP TIME: 20 MINUTES

COOK TIME: 20 MINUTES

NOTE

1. Seniors on a prostate cancer diet should include cooked tomatoes and cruciferous vegetables such as broccoli and cauliflower in their meals.

2. Stay away from red meat and dairy items that are high in fat, and instead choose plant-based proteins like nuts and beans.

3. This meal conforms to these requirements, providing a healthy dinner that encourages better living.

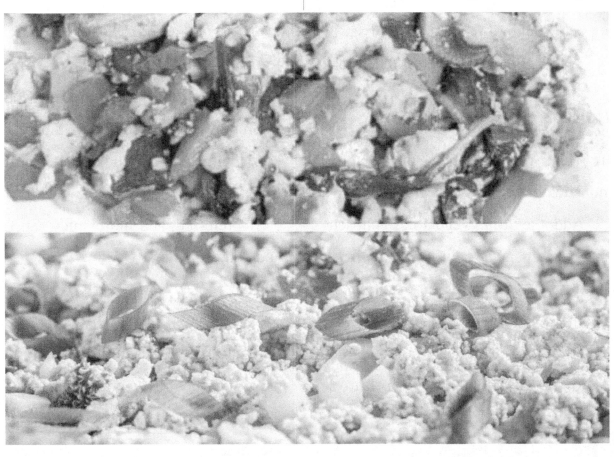

3. Breakfast Burrito With Black Beans Salsa

Start your morning with a tasty and healthy Breakfast Burrito with Black Bean Salsa. The meal is not only tasty, but it also conforms to the diet needs of seniors with prostate cancer, favoring plant-based proteins and antioxidant-rich parts.

INGREDIENTS

- 6 large eggs
- 1 cup of black beans (canned, drained and rinsed)
- 1/2 cup of salsa (choose a low-sodium variety)
- 1/4 cup of shredded cheese (cheddar or a Mexican blend)
- 1/2 teaspoon of cumin
- 1/2 teaspoon of paprika
- Salt and pepper to taste
- 1 tablespoon of olive oil
- 1/2 bell pepper, diced
- 1/4 onion, diced
- 6 8-inch tortillas (whole wheat preferred)

INSTRUCTIONS

1. In a bowl, mix the eggs and season with salt and pepper.

2. Heat the olive oil in a skillet over medium heat. Sauté the bell pepper and onion until tender.

3. Add the eggs to the skillet and scramble until barely set.

4. Heat the black beans in a separate saucepan and season with cumin and paprika.

5. Arrange the tortillas and distribute the scrambled eggs, black beans, salsa, and cheese among them.

6. Roll the tortillas into burritos, tucking in the ends.

7. Serve immediately, or cover with foil to keep warm.

COOKING TIPS

1. For a softer tortilla, warm them slightly before assembling the burritos.

2. Add a handful of spinach or kale to the scramble for an extra nutrient boost.

Nutritional Values Per Serving: Calories: Approximately 350 | Fat: 15g | Carbohydrates: 35g | Protein: 20g

SERVING PORTION: THIS RECIPE MAKES 6 BURRITOS, SERVING 6 PEOPLE.

PREP TIME: 10 MINUTES   COOK TIME: 15 MINUTES

NOTE

1. Black beans are a great source of protein and fiber.

2. The salsa and veggies include antioxidants, which are helpful to general health.

3. Cheese is used sparingly, and you can choose a low-fat one.

4. Whole wheat tortillas are suggested to add fiber.

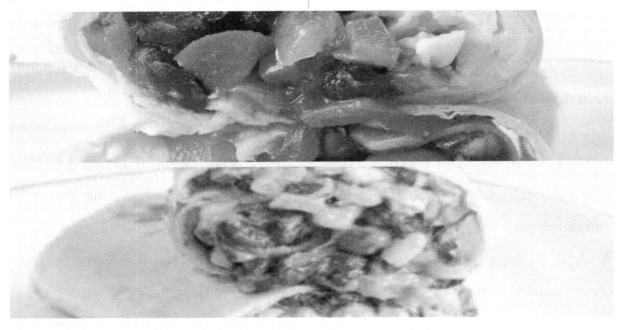

4. Chia Seed Pudding With Mango

Chia Seed Pudding with Mango is a delicious and nutritious treat suitable for seniors. It is high in dietary fiber, protein, and omega-3 fatty acids, making it an ideal option for individuals on a prostate cancer diet. This pudding is simple to prepare and may be served as a breakfast or healthy snack.

INGREDIENTS

- 3 tablespoons of chia seeds
- 1 cup of unsweetened almond milk (or any plant-based milk)
- 1 tablespoon of maple syrup (or, to taste, stevia or monk fruit sweetener)
- 1 teaspoon of vanilla extract
- 1 ripe mango, peeled and diced
- Optional toppings: Additional mango pieces, coconut flakes, or a sprinkle of cinnamon

INSTRUCTIONS

1. In a mixing bowl, mix the chia seeds, almond milk, maple syrup, and vanilla extract. Whisk well until blended.

2. Allow the mixture to settle for about 5 minutes until stirring again to prevent clumping.

3. Cover the bowl and refrigerate for at least 2 hours, preferably overnight until the mixture has a pudding-like consistency.

4. Before serving, mix the pudding again and check for consistency. If it is too thick, add a bit more milk to achieve the required consistency.

5. Serve the pudding in meals or glasses, stacked or topped with fresh, chopped mango and any other desired toppings.

COOKING TIPS

1. For a smoother texture, blend half of the mango and mix it into the pudding.

2. If using frozen mango, thaw it overnight in the fridge or defrost it briefly in the microwave before using.

Nutritional Values Per Serving: Calories: Approximately 200 | Fat: 7g | Carbohydrates: 30g | Protein: 5g | Fiber: 10g

SERVING PORTION: THIS RECIPE SERVES 2.

PREP TIME: 10 MINUTES (PLUS CHILLING TIME)

NOTE

1. Almond milk and chia seeds include beneficial lipids and proteins.

2. Mangoes are abundant in antioxidants, which promote general health.

3. This meal prevents the use of red meat and dairy products, in line with nutritional recommendations for prostate cancer.

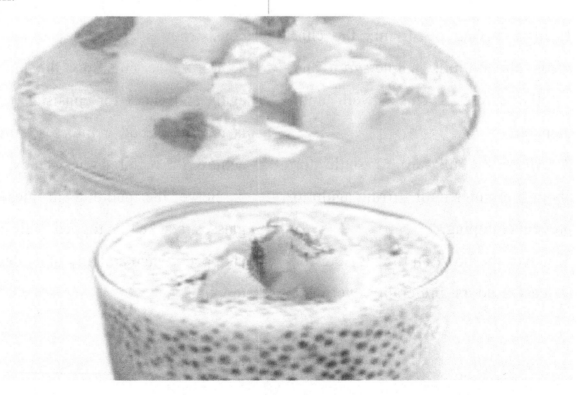

5. Oatmeal With Pecans And Dried Cranberries

Enjoy a warm and soothing cup of oatmeal with pecans and dried cranberries. This recipe is not only comforting, but it also meets the nutritional demands of seniors with prostate cancer. It's high in fiber, antioxidants, and healthy fats, making it a great breakfast alternative.

INGREDIENTS

- 1 cup of old-fashioned oats
- 2 cups of water or milk alternative (such as almond milk)
- 1/4 cup of dried cranberries
- 1/4 cup of pecans, chopped
- 1 tablespoon of maple syrup (optional)
- 1/2 teaspoon of cinnamon
- Pinch of salt

INSTRUCTIONS

1. Heat the water or milk alternative in a medium pot until it boils.

2. Stir in the oats and a bit of salt, and reduce the heat to a simmer.

3. Cook for about 5 minutes, stirring frequently, until the oats have softened and absorbed most of the liquid.

4. Remove from heat and add the cinnamon, dried cranberries, and pecans.

5. If preferred, sweeten with maple syrup and serve warm.

COOKING TIPS

1. To add texture, roast the nuts in a dry pan before mixing them into the oats.

2. If you like a thinner consistency, add extra liquid to suit.

Nutritional Values Per Serving: Calories: Approximately 300 | Fat: 8g | Carbohydrates: 50g | Protein: 6g | Fiber: 7g

SERVING PORTION: THIS RECIPE SERVES 2.

PREP TIME: 5 MINUTES

COOK TIME: 10 MINUTES

NOTE

1. This oatmeal dish is good for a prostate cancer diet because it contains whole grains, nuts, and dried fruits, all of which are high in nutrients and have the potential to improve general health.

2. It's vital to include meals like stewed tomatoes, cruciferous vegetables, and plant-based proteins while limiting red meat and dairy items.

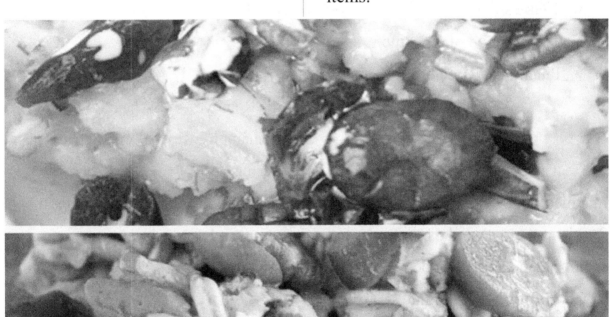

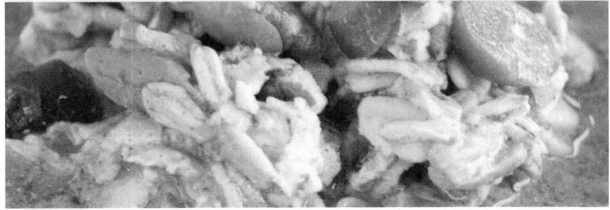

6. Almond Butter Banana Smoothie Bowl

This Almond Butter Banana Smoothie Bowl is a creamy, healthy, and delicious way to start the day. It's high in protein, healthy fats, and fiber, making it a perfect breakfast for seniors, especially those on a prostate cancer diet. The natural sweetness of bananas combined with the richness of almond butter results in a wonderful meal that is both simple to make and good for your health.

INGREDIENTS

- 2 frozen bananas
- 2 tablespoons of almond butter
- 1 tablespoon of ground flaxseed (for added fiber and omega-3s)
- 1/2 teaspoon of cinnamon
- 1/2 cup of unsweetened almond milk (or any plant-based milk of your choice)
- Optional toppings: Sliced banana, almonds, walnuts, sunflower seeds, additional almond butter, or a sprinkle of cinnamon

INSTRUCTIONS

1. Add the frozen bananas, almond butter, ground flaxseed, cinnamon, and almond milk to a blender.

2. Blend on high until the mixture is smooth and creamy.

3. Transfer the smoothie mixture to a bowl.

4. Add any of your preferred toppings for extra texture and nutrition.

COOKING TIPS

1. Make sure the bananas are completely frozen to give the smoothie bowl a thick, ice-cream-like texture.

2. If the smoothie is too thick, add a little extra almond milk to reach the ideal texture.

Nutritional Values Per Serving: Calories: Approximately 370 | Fat: 16g | Carbohydrates: 50g | Protein: 9g | Fiber: 7g

SERVING PORTION: THIS RECIPE SERVES 1.

PREP TIME: 5 MINUTES (JUST BLENDING)

NOTE

1. Almond butter and flaxseed include beneficial fats and proteins.

2. Bananas and cinnamon contain antioxidants, which are helpful to general health.

3. This meal excludes red meat and dairy ingredients, which aligns with prostate cancer diet recommendations.

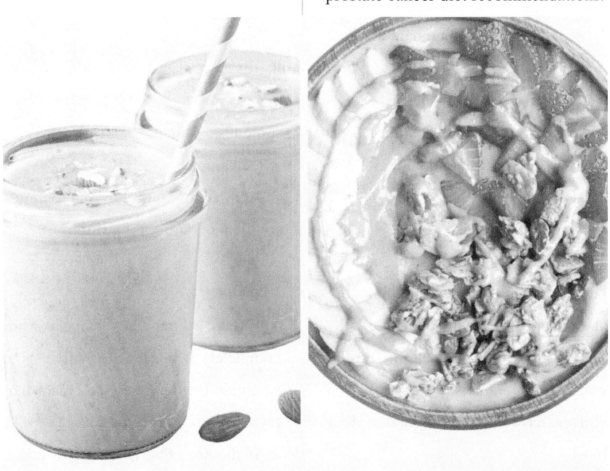

7. Sweet Potato Hash With Turkey Sausage

Sweet Potato Hash with Turkey Sausage is a strong and healthy dish perfect for seniors seeking a well-balanced diet, particularly those fighting prostate cancer. This meal is nutrient-dense, high in protein, and low in saturated fat, making it suitable for prostate health.

INGREDIENTS

- 2 medium sweet potatoes, peeled and diced (about 4 cups)
- 1 tablespoon of olive oil
- 1 pound of turkey sausage, casing removed
- 1 medium onion, diced
- 1 red bell pepper, diced
- 2 cloves of garlic, minced
- 1 teaspoon of smoked paprika
- 1/2 teaspoon of ground cumin
- Salt and pepper, to taste
- 4 large eggs (optional, for topping)
- Fresh parsley, chopped (for garnish)

INSTRUCTIONS

1. Heat your oven to 400°F (200°C).

2. Toss the sweet potatoes with olive oil, salt, and pepper, then lay them out on a baking sheet.

3. Roast for 20-25 minutes, until tender and slightly caramelized.

4. While the sweet potatoes roast, prepare a large pan over medium heat.

5. Cook the turkey sausage in the pan, breaking it up with a spoon, until browned.

6. Place the onion, bell pepper, garlic, smoked paprika, and cumin in the pan with the sausage. Cook for another 5-7 minutes, or until the veggies have softened.

7. When the sweet potatoes are finished, transfer them to the skillet and stir everything together.

8. If preferred, make four wells in the hash and crack one egg into each. Cover the skillet and simmer until the eggs are done to your preference.

9. Just before serving, garnish with fresh parsley.

COOKING TIPS

1. After adding the sweet potatoes, broil the pan for a few minutes to get a crispier hash.

2. You may add more vegetables, like spinach or kale, to this hash to boost its nutritional value.

Nutritional Values Per Serving: Calories: Approximately 350 | Fat: 18g | Carbohydrates: 24g | Protein: 20g

SERVING PORTION: THIS RECIPE SERVES 4.

PREP TIME: 15 MINUTES

COOK TIME: 35 MINUTES

NOTE

1. This meal is excellent for a prostate cancer diet since it contains lean protein from turkey sausage and a variety of veggies.

2. Eat meals high in fiber, antioxidants, and healthy fats while reducing red meat and dairy items.

3. Sweet potatoes are high in fiber and vitamins, and heating them in olive oil improves nutritional absorption.

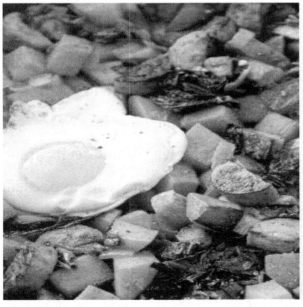 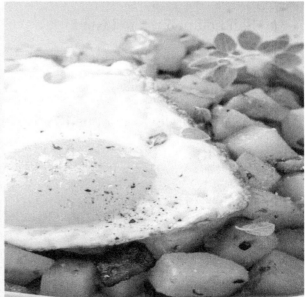

8. Spinach And Feta Omellete

This Spinach and Feta Omelette is a tasty and nutritious option for seniors, particularly those following a prostate cancer diet. It's high in protein, healthy fats, and vitamins, making it an ideal breakfast option.

INGREDIENTS

- 1 teaspoon of olive oil
- 1 cup of baby spinach
- Kosher salt and freshly ground pepper, to taste
- 2 to 3 large eggs
- 1 tablespoon of unsalted butter
- 1/4 cup of crumbled feta cheese (or goat cheese)
- 2 teaspoons of minced fresh chives, for garnish (optional)

INSTRUCTIONS

1. Put an 8-inch omelette pan or shallow skillet, ideally nonstick pan, over medium-high heat.

2. Heat the olive oil, then add the spinach, season with salt and pepper, and toss for one minute until wilted. Transfer to a smaller plate.

3. Crack the eggs into a small bowl and beat them with a fork. Season with salt and pepper.

4. Melt the butter in the same pan, then add the eggs.

5. Cook the eggs, without stirring, until they start to set on the bottom.

6. On one side of the omelette, sprinkle the wilted spinach and crumbled feta.

7. Carefully fold the second half of the omelette over the filling, using a spatula.

8. Cook for another minute, or until the omelette is cooked to your preference.

9. Transfer the omelette to a platter, top it with chives, and serve immediately.

COOKING TIPS

1. For a fluffy omelette, add a dash of milk to the eggs before beating.

2. Use a nonstick pan so the omelette can be easily folded and served.

Nutritional Values Per Serving: Calories: Approximately 300 | Fat: 22g | Carbohydrates: 2g | Protein: 20g

SERVING PORTION: THIS RECIPE SERVES 1.

PREP TIME: 5 MINUTES

COOK TIME: 5 MINUTES

NOTE

1. Seniors on a prostate cancer diet should eat foods strong in fiber, antioxidants, and healthy fats while reducing red meat and dairy.

2. This omelette is a good choice since it contains healthy fats from olive oil and protein from eggs.

3. Cooked veggies, such as spinach, are also helpful.

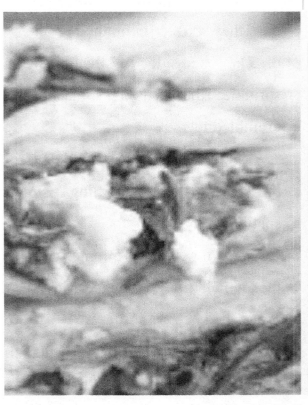 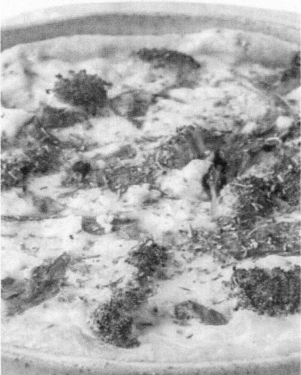

9. Avocado Toast With Poached Egg

Avocado Toast with Poached Egg is a simple and beautiful breakfast that mixes creamy avocado with a delicate poached egg. It's a meal that's not only tasty but also high in nutrients that are good for prostate cancer.

INGREDIENTS

- 1 ripe avocado
- 2 slices of whole-grain bread
- 2 large eggs
- 1 tablespoon of white vinegar (for poaching the eggs)
- Salt and pepper, to taste
- Optional toppings: Chopped herbs, red pepper flakes, or a drizzle of olive oil

INSTRUCTIONS

1. Begin by poaching the eggs. Bring a saucepan of water to a low heat and add the white vinegar.

2. Crack each egg into a small dish and carefully place it in the boiling water, one at a time.

3. Cook for 3–4 minutes for soft yolks and 5–6 minutes for tougher yolks. Using a slotted spoon, take the eggs and drain them on a paper towel.

4. While the eggs are poaching, toast the whole-grain bread to your preferred crispiness.

5. Mash the avocado and season with salt and pepper.

6. Evenly spread the mashed avocado on the toasted bread slices.

7. Top each piece with a poached egg and any other toppings you choose.

COOKING TIPS

8. Before adding the poached eggs, create a gentle vortex in the boiling water.

9. To add flavor, stir together a little lemon juice or zest with the mashed avocado.

Nutritional Values Per Serving: Calories: Approximately 350 | Fat: 20g | Carbohydrates: 30g | Protein: 14g

SERVING PORTION: THIS RECIPE SERVES 2.

PREP TIME: 10 MINUTES

COOK TIME: 10 MINUTES

NOTE

1. This dish is appropriate for a prostate cancer diet since it has avocado's healthful fats and egg' protein.

2. Whole-grain bread contains fiber, and the meal is low in saturated fat.

3. Include a mix of vegetables and fruits, lean meats, and healthy grains, while reducing red meat and high-fat dairy items.

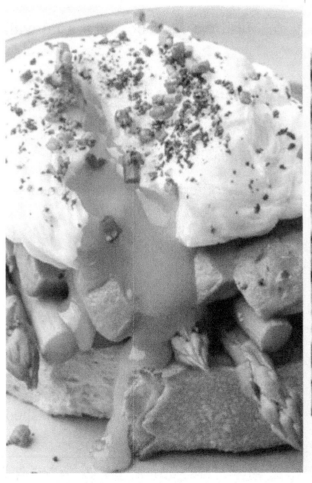
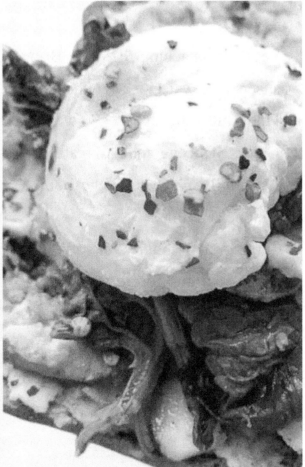

10. Spinach And Mushroom Frittata

Avocado Toast with Poached Egg is a traditional, nutritious breakfast that blends heart-healthy fats from avocado with high-quality protein from eggs. It's a simple yet fulfilling meal that fits well into a prostate cancer diet for seniors, with a focus on nutritious grains, healthy fats, and lean protein sources.

INGREDIENTS

- 1 ripe avocado
- 2 slices of whole-grain bread
- 2 large eggs
- 1 tablespoon of white vinegar (for poaching the eggs)
- Salt and pepper, to taste
- Optional toppings: Chopped herbs, red pepper flakes, or a drizzle of olive oil

INSTRUCTIONS

1. Pour water into a medium pot and heat to a low simmer. Add the white vinegar.

2. Crack each egg into a small bowl and carefully place it in the boiling water, one at a time.

3. Cook for 3–4 minutes for a soft yolk and 5–6 minutes for a harder yolk. Using a slotted spoon, take the eggs and drain them on a paper towel.

4. While the eggs are poaching, toast the whole- grain bread to your preferred crispiness.

5. Mash the avocado in a bowl, then season with salt and pepper.

6. Spread the mashed avocado equally on the toasted bread slices.

7. Top each piece with a poached egg and any other desired toppings.

COOKING TIPS

1. Before adding the poached eggs, create a slight vortex in the boiling water to achieve a good consistency.

2. To add flavor, stir together a little lemon juice or zest with the mashed avocado.

Nutritional Values Per Serving: Calories: Approximately 350 | Fat: 20g | Carbohydrates: 30g | Protein: 14g

SERVING PORTION: THIS RECIPE SERVES 2.

PREP TIME: 10 MINUTES

COOK TIME: 10 MINUTES

NOTE

1. Seniors on a prostate cancer diet should focus on a diet high in vegetables, whole grains, and lean proteins while limiting red meat and dairy items.

2. This meal is suitable since avocados contain healthy fats and eggs contain protein.

3. Whole-grain bread adds fiber to the meal, which is low in saturated fat. It is advantageous to consume a variety of vegetables and fruits, lean proteins, and whole grains while reducing red meat and high-fat dairy products.

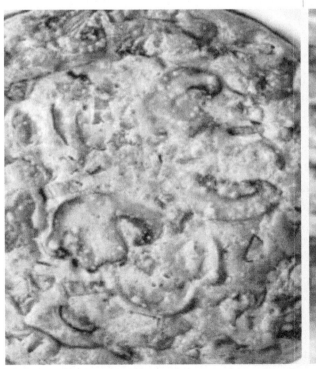
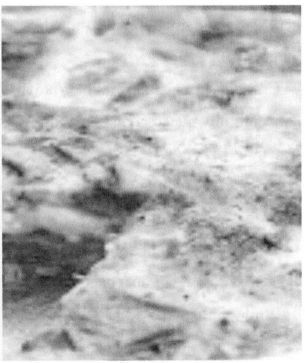

11. Whole Grain Avocado Toast

Whole Grain Avocado Toast is a simple, healthy, and varied breakfast choice that is ideal for seniors. It is high in heart-healthy monounsaturated fats, fiber, and important nutrients, which fit with prostate cancer dietary guidelines.

INGREDIENTS

- 2 slices of whole-grain bread
- 1 ripe avocado
- Salt and pepper, to taste
- Optional toppings: Sliced tomatoes, radishes, or a sprinkle of sesame seeds

INSTRUCTIONS

1. Toast the whole grain bread slices to your desired crispiness.

2. Cut the avocado in half, remove the pit, and spoon the flesh into a bowl as the bread toasts.

3. Using a fork, mash the avocado until creamy. Season with salt and pepper.

4. Evenly spread the mashed avocado across the toasted bread.

5. Add any additional toppings for taste and nutrition.

COOKING TIPS

1. Squeeze some lemon juice over the mashed avocado for extra flavor.

2. If you want a little heat, add a sprinkle of chili flakes to your toast.

Nutritional Values Per Serving: Calories: Approximately 250 | Fat: 15g | Carbohydrates: 24g | Protein: 6g

SERVING PORTION: THIS RECIPE SERVES 1.

PREP TIME: 5 MINUTES   COOK TIME: 5 MINUTES

NOTE

1. Eat foods rich in antioxidants and good fats while limiting saturated fats found in red meat and dairy products.

2. Whole-grain bread is rich in fiber, and avocados have healthy fats that promote heart and prostate health.

12. Sautéed Chard with Feta and Egg Breakfast Toast

Sautéed Chard with Feta and Egg Breakfast Toast is a healthy and tasty way to start the day. It contains dark leafy greens that are high in carotenoids, which have been found to reduce the growth of some types of cancer cells, making it a good choice for a prostate cancer diet.

INGREDIENTS

- 1 slice whole grain bread
- 2 large chard leaves, chopped
- 1 tsp. of olive oil
- 1 tsp. of feta cheese
- 1 hard-boiled egg, thinly sliced

INSTRUCTIONS

1. Toast the bread to your preferred level of crispiness.

2. Sauté chopped chard in olive oil until tender and reduced by ¾ size.

3. Spread the sautéed chard on top of the bread.

4. Sprinkle with feta cheese.

5. Top with a thinly sliced, hard-boiled egg.

COOKING TIPS

1. If desired, you may substitute spinach or kale for the chard.

2. Add a squeeze of lemon, minced garlic, or crushed red pepper flakes to the chard while sautéing for more flavor.

Nutritional Values Per Serving: Calories: Approx. 220 | Cholesterol: 190 mg | Carbohydrates: 15g | Protein: 7g | Fiber: 3g | Sodium: 250mg | Sugar: 3g

SERVING PORTION: THIS RECIPE MAKES 1 SERVING.

PREP TIME: 5 MINUTES   COOK TIME: 10 MINUTES

NOTE: For seniors on a prostate cancer diet, it's essential to integrate stewed tomatoes and cruciferous vegetables like broccoli and cauliflower into meals, minimize fat from red meat and dairy products, and opt for plant-based proteins like nuts and beans.

13. Southwest Vegetable Frittata

This Southwest Vegetable Frittata is a tasty and health-conscious option for seniors, especially those following a prostate cancer diet. It's filled with veggies, black beans, and spices, making it a healthy meal that's both filling and good for your health.

INGREDIENTS

- 1 red bell pepper, seeded and chopped
- 1 green pepper, seeded and chopped
- 1 jalapeno, seeded and chopped
- 1 onion, chopped
- 8 oz. mushrooms, sliced
- 1 can of black beans, drained
- 1 can of diced tomatoes
- 8 eggs
- 1/3 cup milk (or a milk alternative)
- Salt and pepper, to taste
- 2 tablespoons olive oil
- 1/2 cup cheese (use a reduced-fat variety if preferred)
- Optional: Hot sauce and parsley garnish

INSTRUCTIONS

1. Preheat the broiler on low.

2. Prepare all of your ingredients and ensure they are ready to use.

3. In a medium pitcher, mix the eggs, milk, salt, and pepper to taste.

4. Preheat a big cast-iron skillet to medium-high heat. Add olive oil.

5. Simmer the onions and peppers for 5 minutes, stirring regularly.

6. Add the mushrooms and sauté until they start to brown.

7. Add the drained beans and canned tomatoes. Continue to cook for a few minutes.

8. Add the egg mixture and lower the heat to medium-low.

9. Once the mixture begins to boil, sprinkle it with cheese and broil in the top third of the oven.

10. Broil until the eggs have set and the cheese is melted and brown.

COOKING TIPS

1. Omit the cheese or substitute a dairy-free cheese for a dairy-free version.

2. To boost fiber content, add a handful of spinach or kale to the vegetable mixture.

Nutritional Values Per Serving: Calories: Approximately 300 | Fat: 18g | Carbohydrates: 15g | Protein: 20g

SERVING PORTION: THIS RECIPE YIELDS 4-6 SERVINGS.

PREP TIME: 15 MINUTES

COOK TIME: 30 MINUTES

NOTE

1. For seniors on a prostate cancer diet, it's essential to include cooked tomatoes and cruciferous vegetables like broccoli and cauliflower in many of their weekly meals, limit fat from red meat and dairy products, and choose plant-based proteins such as nuts and beans.

2. This frittata recipe follows these principles, providing a healthy and tasty meal.

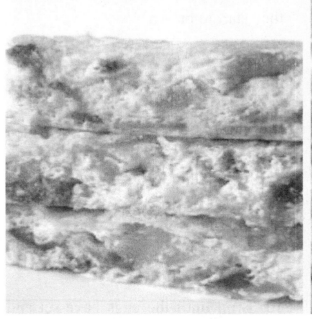
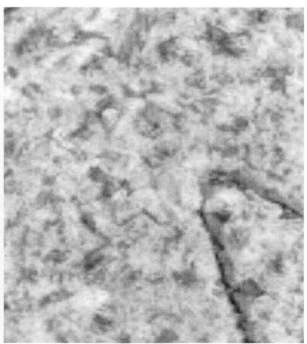

14. Strawberry Chia Smoothie

This Strawberry Chia Smoothie is both refreshing and healthy, making it ideal for seniors. It includes antioxidants from strawberries and omega-3 fatty acids from chia seeds, making it a good choice for those on a prostate cancer diet.

INGREDIENTS

- 1 cup of frozen strawberries to ensure a creamy and thick smoothie texture.
- 1 ripe banana for natural sweetness.
- 1/2 cup of Greek yogurt for a protein boost.
- 1 cup of unsweetened almond milk or any other milk of your choice.
- 1 tablespoon of chia seeds for added texture and nutrients.
- 1/2 teaspoon of vanilla extract for flavor enhancement.

INSTRUCTIONS

1. Add the frozen strawberries, banana, Greek yogurt, and almond milk to a blender.

2. Blend on high until the mixture is completely smooth.

3. Combine the chia seeds and vanilla essence, then pulse a few times to combine them.

4. Transfer the smoothie to a glass and let it sit for a few minutes to allow the chia seeds to swell and thicken the liquid.

COOKING TIPS

1. For the finest chia seed smoothie results, add the chia seeds last, after blending the other ingredients.

2. If you don't have frozen strawberries, put fresh strawberries and a handful of ice in the blender before adding the chia seeds.

Nutritional Values Per Serving: Calories: Approximately 300 | Fat: 9g | Carbohydrates: 44g | Protein: 14g | Fiber: 10g

SERVING PORTION: THIS RECIPE MAKES 1 SERVING.

PREP TIME: 5 MINUTES (JUST BLENDING)

1. For seniors on a prostate cancer diet, it is critical to prioritize foods high in antioxidants and good fats while limiting saturated fats from red meat and dairy.

2. This smoothie has healthy fats from chia seeds and protein from Greek yogurt.

3. Strawberries include fiber and antioxidants, and the drink is low in saturated fat.

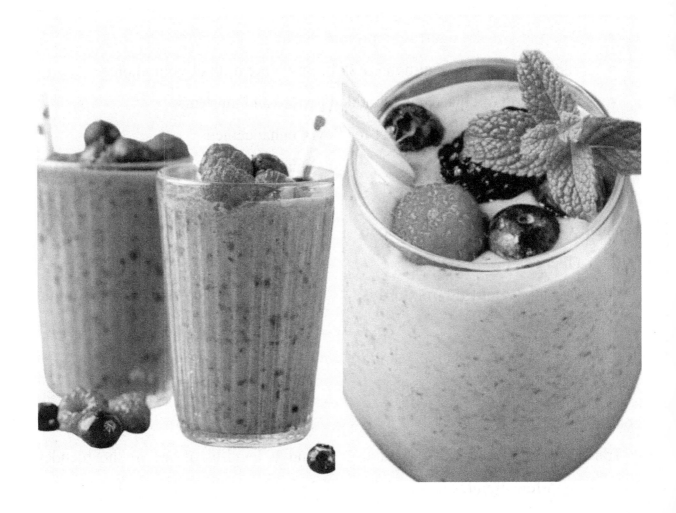

15. Ricotta, Basil, and Strawberry Toast

Ricotta, Basil, and Strawberry Toast is a refreshing and tasty meal that mixes ricotta's creamy texture with the sweetness of strawberries and an enticing touch of basil. It's a simple yet complex breakfast or snack that's not only delicious but also follows prostate-healthy nutritional advice.

INGREDIENTS

- 4 slices of thick, crusty bread
- 1/2 cup of full-fat ricotta cheese
- 1 rounded teaspoon of honey
- Zest of 1/2 lemon
- 12 large strawberries, sliced
- 8 leaves of fresh basil, chopped

FOR BALSAMIC REDUCTION

- 1/2 cup of balsamic vinegar
- 1/4 cup of honey

INSTRUCTIONS

1. In a small saucepan, combine balsamic vinegar and honey and simmer for about 10 minutes, until the volume is reduced by half.

2. On a grill or grill pan, toast the bread on both sides.

3. Mix the ricotta, honey, and lemon zest.

4. Top the grilled bread with the ricotta mixture, strawberries, and basil.

5. Pour with balsamic reduction and serve immediately.

COOKING TIPS

1. If you like, you may add a drizzle of honey instead of the balsamic for an added flavor boost.

2. For the greatest tasting reduction, use high-quality balsamic vinegar.

Nutritional Values Per Serving: Calories: Approximately 300 | Fat: 9g | Carbohydrates: 44g | Protein: 14g | Fiber: 5g

SERVING PORTION: THIS RECIPE MAKES 4 SERVINGS.

PREP TIME: 10 MINUTES

COOK TIME: 10 MINUTES

NOTE

1. Seniors on a prostate cancer diet should consume foods high in antioxidants and good fats while limiting saturated fats from red meat and dairy products.

2. This toast is good since it contains healthy fats from ricotta and antioxidants from strawberries.

3. Whole-grain bread contains fiber, and the meal is low in saturated fat.

4. It is helpful to eat a variety of vegetables and fruits, lean proteins, and whole grains, while reducing red meat and high-fat dairy products.

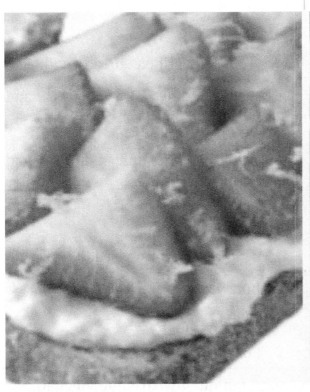
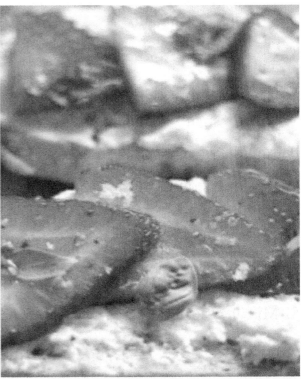

CHAPTER 4: LUNCH DIET FOR PROSTATE CANCER

1. Salmon and Veggie Egg Muffins

Salmon & Veggie Egg Muffins are a quick, easy, adaptable, and healthy meal that adheres to the nutritional requirements for prostate cancer prevention and survival. They are high in protein, veggies, and whole grains, making them a great option for any time of day.

INGREDIENTS

- Nonstick cooking spray
- 2 tsp. of extra-virgin olive oil
- 1/2 red bell pepper, cut into 1/2-inch dice
- 2 cups of baby spinach, roughly chopped and packed
- 2 green onions, trimmed, sliced, and chopped
- 5 large eggs
- One 2.6-ounce of pouch wild-caught pink salmon in extra-virgin olive oil, flaked
- 1/2 cup of shredded reduced-fat Cheddar cheese
- 1/4 cup of fresh basil, finely chopped
- Kosher salt and black pepper, to taste
- 100% whole-grain bread, toasted
- Optional spreads for toast: Smashed avocado, olive oil, nut butter, hummus, butter substitute

INSTRUCTIONS

1. Set the oven to 350°F. Lightly spray a 6-cup muffin tin with nonstick cooking spray and set aside.

2. Heat the oil in a nonstick skillet over medium-high heat. Cook the peppers, turning regularly, until tender, approximately 5 minutes. If the peppers start to burn, turn the heat down to medium.

3. Cook, stirring regularly, until the spinach and onions are wilted, about 2 minutes. Allow it to cool a little bit.

4. Crack the eggs into a large bowl. Mix until well blended.

5. Stir in the salmon, cheese, basil, cooked veggies, salt, and pepper until well blended.

COOKING TIPS

1. You may substitute tuna for salmon if you like.

6. Divide the mixture evenly among the prepared muffin cups using a 1/3 measuring cup.

7. Bake for 18 minutes, or until the eggs have set.

2. To avoid premature frying of the eggs, allow the veggies to cool somewhat before adding them to the eggs.

Nutritional Values Per Serving: Calories: Approx. 280 | Cholesterol: 325 mg | Carbohydrates: 8 g | Protein: 22 g | Fiber: 2 g | Sodium: 350 mg | Sugar: 2 g

SERVING PORTION: THIS RECIPE MAKES 3 SERVINGS (2 EGG MUFFINS PER SERVING).

PREP TIME: 10 MINUTES   COOK TIME: 18 MINUTES

NOTE: For seniors on a prostate cancer diet, it's essential to include stewed tomatoes and cruciferous vegetables like broccoli and cauliflower in many of their weekly meals, limit fat from red meat and dairy products, and choose plant-based proteins like nuts and beans.

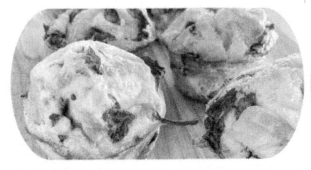
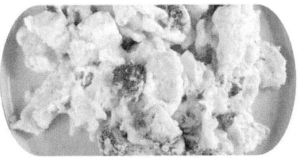

2. Walnut Tomato Sauce with Zucchini Lasagna Noodles

This Walnut Tomato Sauce with Zucchini Lasagna Noodles puts a modern spin on traditional lasagna, using zucchini noodles and a rich tomato sauce filled with the benefits of walnuts, creating a healthy meal that promotes a prostate cancer diet.

INGREDIENTS

- Zucchini "Lasagna Noodles"
- 4 small zucchini squashes

FOR THE SAUCE

- 1 tablespoon of extra virgin olive oil
- 1 medium onion, finely diced
- 3 cloves garlic, minced
- 2 stalks celery, finely chopped
- 5 ounces (about 2 cups) of mushrooms, thinly sliced
- 1 32-ounce jar of marinara sauce
- 2 tablespoons of tomato paste
- 1 tablespoon of soy sauce

- 1/2 cup of red wine
- 1 tablespoon of Italian seasoning blend
- 1/2 teaspoon of black pepper
- 1/4 teaspoon of salt (optional)
- 1 ½ cups of ground walnuts, divided

FILLING

- 1 cup of shredded plant-based cheese (or dairy-based cheese, if preferred)

GARNISH

- 2 tablespoons of chopped Italian parsley

INSTRUCTIONS

1. Cut zucchini horizontally into long, thin slices (5 horizontal slices per squash). To soak up any excess moisture, place on paper towels.

2. In a Dutch oven or big saucepan, heat the olive oil over medium heat.

Sauté onion, garlic, and celery for 3 minutes, stirring constantly.

3. Add the mushrooms and sauté for another 2 minutes.

4. Mix in the marinara sauce, tomato paste, soy sauce, red wine, Italian

spice, black pepper, and salt (optional). Cover and boil for 10-15 minutes, or until the mixture thickens and the veggies are cooked.

5. Heat the oven to 350°F (175° C). Spray a 13-by-9-inch baking dish with nonstick cooking spray.

6. Arrange one-third of the zucchini slices at the bottom of the dish. Top with one-third of the walnut tomato sauce and 1/3 cup shredded cheese. Repeat the layering two more times.

7. Bake uncovered for 40 minutes. Sprinkle the remaining ¼ cup ground walnuts on top and broil for 2 minutes until golden.

COOKING TIPS

1. Store walnuts in the refrigerator or freezer to preserve their freshness and quality.

2. For a "meaty" texture, ensure the walnuts are finely ground but not overly processed to a flour texture.

Nutritional Values Per Serving: Calories: 282 | Fat: 17g | Sodium: 231 mg | Carbohydrates: 26g | Fiber: 5g | Sugars: 12g | Protein: 5g

SERVING PORTION: THIS RECIPE SERVES 8.

PREP TIME: 20 MINUTES

COOK TIME: 1 HOUR, 5 MINUTES

NOTE: For seniors on a prostate cancer diet, it's important to include cooked tomatoes and cruciferous vegetables like broccoli and cauliflower in their meals, limit fat from red meat and dairy products, and opt for plant-based proteins like nuts and beans.

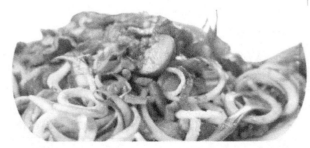
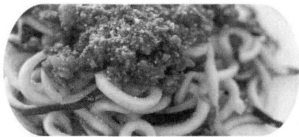

3. Shrimp Salad with Sun-Dried Tomato Vinaigrette

This shrimp salad with sun-dried tomato vinaigrette is a light and flavorful dish ideal for seniors. It is high in protein and antioxidants, making it an ideal choice for those on a prostate cancer diet. The sun-dried tomato vinaigrette has a tangy, robust flavor that compliments the shrimp perfectly.

INGREDIENTS

FOR THE SALAD

- 1 pound of cooked medium shrimp, peeled and deveined
- 5 cups of mixed greens (such as arugula, spinach, and romaine)
- 1/2 cup of cherry tomatoes, halved
- 1/4 cup of red onion, thinly sliced
- 1/4 cup of kalamata olives, pitted and halved
- 1/4 cup of crumbled feta cheese

FOR THE SUN-DRIED TOMATO VINAIGRETTE

- 1/3 cup of sun-dried tomatoes in oil, drained and chopped
- 2 tablespoons of red wine vinegar
- 1 tablespoon of Dijon mustard
- 1 garlic clove, minced
- 1/2 cup of extra virgin olive oil
- Salt and pepper, to taste

INSTRUCTIONS

1. In a large salad bowl, combine the mixed greens, cherry tomatoes, red onion, olives, and feta cheese.

2. In a blender or food processor, combine the sun-dried tomatoes, red wine vinegar, Dijon mustard, and garlic until smooth.

3. With the blender running, gently add the olive oil until the vinaigrette is emulsified. Season with salt and pepper, to taste.

4. Add the cooked shrimp to the salad and pour with the sun-dried tomato vinaigrette. Toss lightly to mix.

5. Serve immediately, topped with more feta cheese if preferred.

COOKING TIPS

1. To get the most flavor out of the vinaigrette, let it rest for about an hour before serving.

2. If you like a less tangy dressing, reduce the vinegar and add a teaspoon of honey to the vinaigrette.

Nutritional Values Per Serving: Calories: Approximately 350 | Fat: 22g | Carbohydrates: 8g | Protein: 25g | Fiber: 2g

SERVING PORTION: THIS RECIPE SERVES 4.

PREP TIME: 15 MINUTES

NOTE

1. Seniors on a prostate cancer diet should prioritize foods strong in antioxidants and good fats while limiting saturated fats found in red meat and dairy items.

2. This salad is suitable as it includes lean protein from shrimp and healthy fats from olive oil. The mixed greens provide fiber and antioxidants, and the dish is low in saturated fat.

3. Including a variety of vegetables and fruits, lean proteins, and whole grains is beneficial, while limiting red meat and high-fat dairy products is recommended

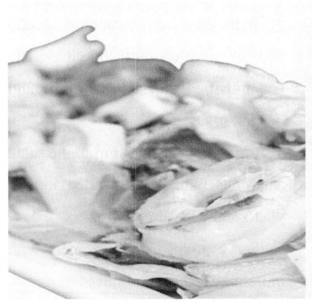
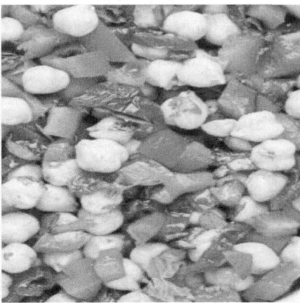

4. Grilled Portobello Mushroom Salad

Grilled Portobello Mushroom Salad is a filling yet light meal, perfect for seniors. It's a tasty and nutritious meal that adheres to prostate health dietary guidelines, with veggies, healthy fats, and plant-based proteins.

INGREDIENTS

- 4 large portobello mushrooms
- 1/2 cup of balsamic vinegar
- 1/4 cup of olive oil
- 1 tablespoon of honey
- 2 garlic of cloves, minced
- 1/2 teaspoon of ground black pepper
- 1 head romaine lettuce, chopped
- 10 cherry tomatoes, halved
- 1 avocado, peeled, pitted, and diced
- 4 ounces of goat cheese

INSTRUCTIONS

1. In a medium bowl, combine the balsamic vinegar, olive oil, honey, black pepper, and garlic.

2. Marinate the mushrooms for at least 15 minutes, stirring them regularly.

3. Preheat the grill to medium.

4. Grill the mushrooms for about 5 minutes per side, or until tender.

5. In a large salad, combine romaine lettuce, cherry tomatoes, avocado, and goat cheese.

6. Slice the grilled mushrooms and mix them into the salad.

7. Serve with your preferred dressing or use the leftover marinade as a dressing.

COOKING TIPS

1. If you have time, marinate the mushrooms for longer to improve the flavors.

2. If you do not have a grill, sauté the mushrooms in a grill pan over medium heat on the stove.

Nutritional Values Per Serving: Calories: Approximately 250 | Fat: 20g | Carbohydrates: 18g | Protein: 8g | Fiber: 5g

SERVING PORTION: THIS RECIPE SERVES 4.

PREP TIME: 20 MINUTES (INCLUDING MARINATING TIME)

COOK TIME: 10 MINUTES

NOTE: For seniors on a prostate cancer diet, it is critical to include stewed tomatoes and cruciferous vegetables such as broccoli and cauliflower in many of their weekly meals, limit fat from red meat and dairy products, and choose plant-based proteins such as nuts and beans.

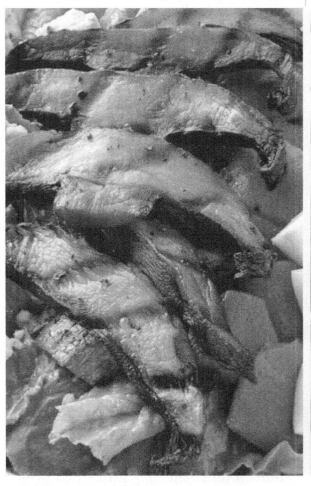 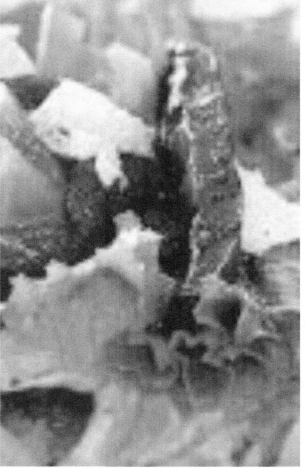

5. Lentil And Vegetable Soup

Lentil and Vegetable Soup is a nourishing, calming dish perfect for seniors. It's high in nutrients, fiber, and protein from lentils and a variety of veggies, making it an ideal choice for those on a prostate cancer diet.

INGREDIENTS

- 1/4 cup of extra virgin olive oil
- 1 medium yellow or white onion, chopped
- 2 carrots, peeled and chopped
- 4 garlic cloves, pressed or minced
- 2 teaspoons of ground cumin
- 1 teaspoon of curry powder
- 1/2 teaspoon of dried thyme
- 1 large can (28 ounces) of diced tomatoes, lightly drained
- 1 cup of brown or green lentils, picked over and rinsed
- 4 cups of vegetable broth
- 2 cups of water
- 1 teaspoon of salt, more to taste
- Pinch of red pepper flakes

INSTRUCTIONS

1. In a large saucepan, warm the olive oil over medium heat. Once heated, add the onion and carrot and cook for 5 minutes, or until softened.

2. Add the garlic, cumin, curry powder, and thyme. Cook until fragrant, approximately 30 seconds.

3. Add the diced tomatoes and cook for a few minutes more, stirring often.

4. Combine the lentils, broth, and water. Season with salt and a sprinkle of red pepper flakes.

5. Bring the soup to a boil, then partially cover and decrease the heat to a low simmer.

6. Cook for 25-30 minutes, or until the lentils are cooked but retain their shape.

7. Add 2 cups of the soup to a blender. Secure the top and puree until smooth. Pour the pureed soup back into the pot. (Alternatively, use an immersion blender to partly mix the soup directly in the saucepan.)

8. Taste and add additional salt as needed. Serve hot.

COOKING TIPS

1. Just before serving, toss in a splash of olive oil or a pat of butter for more texture and richness.

2. If you want a thinner soup, add a bit more water or broth until you achieve the desired consistency.

Nutritional Values Per Serving: Calories: Approximately 250 | Fat: 7g | Carbohydrates: 38g | Protein: 14g | Fiber: 15g

SERVING PORTION: THIS RECIPE YIELDS 4 SERVINGS.

PREP TIME: 10 MINUTES

COOK TIME: 45 MINUTES

NOTE: For seniors on a prostate cancer diet, it's essential to include stewed tomatoes and cruciferous vegetables like broccoli and cauliflower in many of their weekly meals, limit fat from red meat and dairy products, and choose plant-based proteins like nuts and beans.

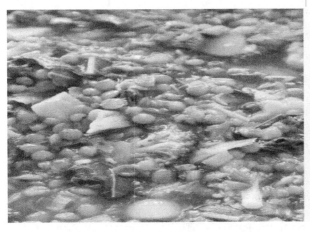
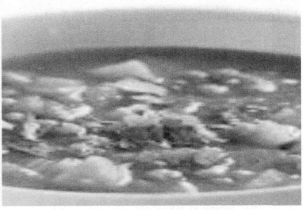

6. Brown Rice Bowl With Teriyaki Salmon

This Brown Rice Bowl with Teriyaki Salmon is a nutritious and delicious dish that combines salmon's high omega-3 fatty acid content with the fiber-rich whole grain of brown rice. It's a well-balanced dinner that's both delicious and in line with prostate health recommended diets.

INGREDIENTS

- 4 salmon fillets (about 6 ounces each)
- 1/4 cup of low-sodium soy sauce or coconut aminos
- 2 tablespoons of honey
- 1 tablespoon of rice vinegar
- 1 teaspoon of minced garlic
- 1 teaspoon of minced ginger
- 1 teaspoon of sesame oil
- 2 cups of cooked brown rice
- 1 avocado, sliced
- 1 cucumber, thinly sliced
- 1 carrot, julienned
- 1/2 cup of edamame beans, shelled and cooked
- Sesame seeds for garnish

INSTRUCTIONS

1. In a mixing bowl, combine soy sauce, honey, rice vinegar, garlic, ginger, and sesame oil to make the teriyaki marinade.

2. Place the salmon fillets in the marinade and refrigerate for at least 30 minutes.

3. Preheat your grill or grill pan to medium heat.

4. Remove the salmon from the marinade and grill for about 4 minutes per side, or until done to your preference.

5. Divide the cooked brown rice into four meals.

6. Garnish each dish with grilled salmon fillets, avocado slices, cucumber, carrot, and edamame beans.

7. Pour with the remaining teriyaki sauce and finish with sesame seeds.

COOKING TIPS

1. Marinate the salmon overnight to give it a stronger taste.

2. To keep the salt content low, use low-sodium soy sauce or coconut aminos.

Nutritional Values Per Serving: Calories: Approximately 500 | Fat: 22g | Carbohydrates: 45g | Protein: 35g | Fiber: 6g

SERVING PORTION: THIS RECIPE SERVES 4.

PREP TIME: 10 MINUTES (PLUS MARINATING TIME)

COOK TIME: 8 MINUTES

NOTE: Seniors on a prostate cancer diet need to eat foods high in antioxidants and good fats while avoiding saturated fats from red meat and dairy products. This meal has healthy fats from salmon and avocado, as well as entire carbohydrates from brown rice.

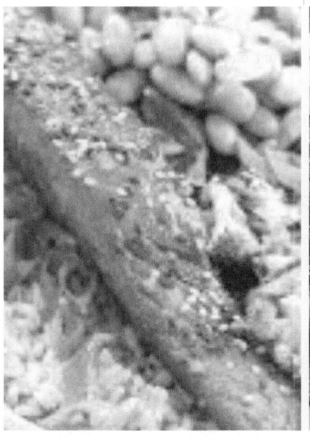 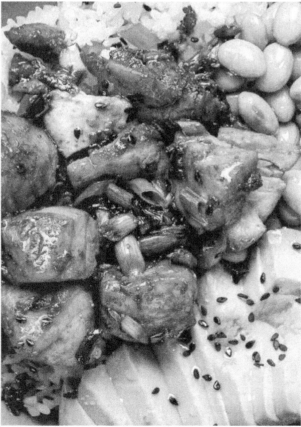

7. Broccoli And Cheddar Stuffed Baked Potatoes

Broccoli & Cheddar Stuffed Baked Potatoes are a satisfying and healthy dish that blends the creamy smoothness of cheddar cheese with the health benefits of broccoli. This meal is ideal for seniors on a prostate cancer diet.

INGREDIENTS

- 4 large russet potatoes
- 1 tablespoon of olive oil
- 1/2 teaspoon of garlic powder
- 1/2 teaspoon of onion powder
- Salt and pepper to taste
- 2 cups of broccoli florets, steamed and chopped
- 1/2 cup of low-fat milk
- 1/4 cup of Greek yogurt
- 1 cup of shredded cheddar cheese, plus more for topping
- 1/4 cup of green onions, chopped

INSTRUCTIONS

1. Heat your oven to 400°F (200°C).

2. Rinse the potatoes and poke them many times with a fork.

3. Coat the potatoes with olive oil, garlic powder, onion powder, salt, and pepper.

4. Place the potatoes on a baking pan and bake for 50-60 minutes, or until well cooked.

5. Cut the potatoes in half lengthwise, then scoop out the insides, leaving a thin layer of potato.

6. In a bowl, mash the scooped potato with the milk and Greek yogurt until smooth.

7. Add the steamed broccoli, cheddar cheese, and green onion.

8. Spoon the mixture back into the potato skins and sprinkle with more cheddar cheese.

9. Bake for another 15-20 minutes, or until the cheese is melted and bubbling.

COOKING TIPS

1. Baking the potatoes directly on the oven rack creates a crispier skin.

2. Use low-fat cheddar cheese to cut the total fat content.

Nutritional Values Per Serving: Calories: Approximately 350 | Fat: 12g | Carbohydrates: 49g | Protein: 15g | Fiber: 4g

SERVING PORTION: THIS RECIPE SERVES 4.

PREP TIME: 10 MINUTES

COOK TIME: 1 HOUR, 10 MINUTES

NOTE: For seniors on a prostate cancer diet, it's essential to include stewed tomatoes and cruciferous vegetables like broccoli and cauliflower into many of their weekly meals, limit fat from red meat and dairy products, and choose plant-based proteins such as nuts and beans.

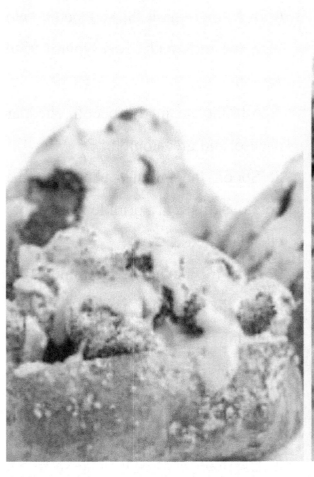
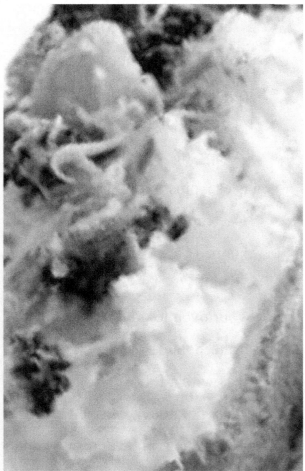

8. Chickpea And Spinach Stew

Chickpea and Spinach Stew is a filling and healthy recipe ideal for seniors. It has a high concentration of plant-based proteins, fiber, and vitamins and minerals. This stew is especially good for those on a prostate cancer diet since it is low in saturated fat and high in nutrient-dense components.

INGREDIENTS

- 2 cans (15 ounces each) of low-sodium chickpeas, rinsed and divided
- 1 tablespoon of olive oil
- 1 medium onion, chopped (1 cup)
- 2 medium carrots, diced (3/4 cup)
- 4 cloves garlic, minced
- 3 tablespoons of tomato paste
- 1 (32 ounce) carton of low-sodium vegetable broth (4 cups)
- 1/4 teaspoon of ground pepper
- 1/8 teaspoon of salt
- 3 cups of fresh spinach (or frozen if preferred)

INSTRUCTIONS

1. Using a fork or potato masher, mash one can of chickpeas. Set aside.

2. Heat the oil in a big saucepan over medium-high heat. Add the carrots, onion, and garlic. Cook, stirring often, until softened and aromatic, 3 to 4 minutes.

3. Add tomato paste and heat for another 30 seconds.

4. Add the vegetable broth, both mashed and whole chickpeas, pepper, and salt to the saucepan. Cover and bring to a simmer.

5. Reduce the heat to medium and simmer, covered, for approximately 10 minutes, or until the veggies are soft and the flavors have combined.

6. Cook until the spinach is wilted, about 2 minutes.

COOKING TIPS

1. If using frozen spinach, be sure to defrost and drain thoroughly before adding it to the stew.

2. To make a thicker stew, combine a piece of it and then stir it back in.

Nutritional Values Per Serving: Calories: Approximately 250 | Fat: 4g | Carbohydrates: 40g | Protein: 14g | Fiber: 10g

SERVING PORTION: THIS RECIPE YIELDS 4 SERVINGS.

PREP TIME: 10 MINUTES

COOK TIME: 20 MINUTES

NOTE : Seniors on a prostate cancer diet should consume foods high in antioxidants and good fats, while limiting saturated fats from red meat and dairy products. This stew is ideal since it contains healthy fats from olive oil and plant-based protein from chickpeas. Spinach contains fiber and antioxidants, and the meal is low in saturated fat. Including a range of vegetables and fruits, lean proteins, and whole grains is advantageous, but minimizing red meat and high-fat dairy items is suggested.

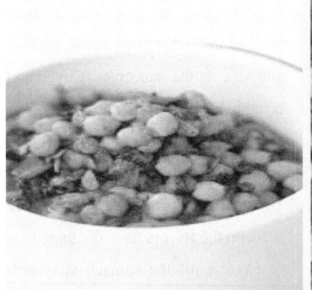
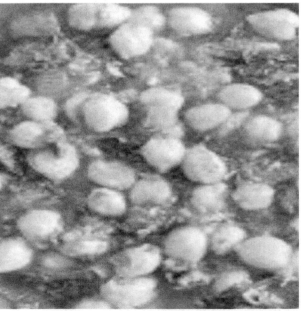

9. Barley and Vegetable Stir-Fry

Barley and Vegetable Stir-Fry is a colorful and nutritious recipe that is ideal for seniors. It's high in fiber from barley and has plenty of nutrients from veggies. This stir-fry is simple to make and can be modified with your favorite veggies.

INGREDIENTS

- 1/2 cup of pearl barley
- 2 teaspoons of canola oil
- 1 medium red onion, diced
- 1 red bell pepper, seeded and diced
- 2 ounces of fresh shiitake mushrooms, stemmed and chopped
- 8 snow peas, cut lengthwise into thin strips
- 2 scallions, green and white parts, chopped
- 3/4 teaspoon of ginger, grated, peeled, according to taste
- 1/2 cup of orange juice
- 1 tablespoon of reduced-sodium soy sauce or teriyaki sauce
- Salt & freshly ground black pepper, to taste

INSTRUCTIONS

1. In a big saucepan, bring 2 cups of water to a boil. Add barley. When the liquid returns to a boil, decrease the heat, cover, and cook for 30 to 40 minutes, or until the barley is nearly tender.

2. Heat the oil in a medium nonstick pan over high heat. Stir-fry the onion and red pepper for one minute.

3. Stir in the mushrooms and cook for 1 minute, or until they seem moist.

4. Stir in the snow peas, scallions, and ginger, cooking for 15 seconds.

5. Stir in cooked barley, orange juice, teriyaki sauce, and salt and pepper to taste. Cook the barley until it is well heated.

COOKING TIPS

1. Feel free to add more veggies, such as broccoli, carrots, or spinach, to boost nutrients.

2. If you want a gluten-free alternative, use gluten-free soy sauce or tamari.

Nutritional Values Per Serving: Calories: Approximately 200 | Fat: 4g | Carbohydrates: 37g | Protein: 6g | Fiber: 9g

SERVING PORTION: THIS RECIPE SERVES 4.

PREP TIME: 10 MINUTES (EXCLUDING BARLEY COOKING TIME)

COOK TIME: 15 MINUTES

NOTE: Seniors on a prostate cancer diet should prioritize plant-based meals, add stewed tomatoes and cruciferous vegetables such as broccoli and cauliflower into many of their weekly meals, and limit their intake of red meat and dairy products. This meal allows you to enjoy a range of veggies and healthy grains, both of which are good for your prostate.

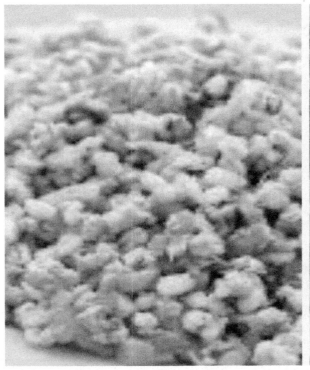
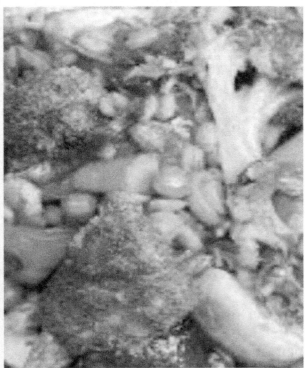

10. Quinoa Salad with Grilled Chicken

Quinoa Salad with Grilled Chicken is a clean and nutritious dish that is ideal for seniors dealing with prostate cancer. It contains nutrients that are proven to promote health and well-being, with an emphasis on anti-inflammatory and antioxidant-rich foods.

INGREDIENTS

- 1 cup of quinoa (uncooked)
- 2 chicken breasts (approximately 6-8 ounces each)
- 1 cup of cherry tomatoes, halved
- 1 cup of cucumber, diced
- 1/2 cup of red onion, finely chopped
- 1/4 cup of kalamata olives, sliced
- 1/4 cup of feta cheese, crumbled
- 2 tbsp. of extra virgin olive oil
- Juice of 1 lemon
- Salt and pepper, to taste
- Mixed greens, for serving (optional)

INSTRUCTIONS

1. To begin, rinse the quinoa in cold water to remove its bitter natural covering.

2. Cook the quinoa according to package instructions, generally for approximately 15 minutes, until fluffy and water is absorbed. Allow it to cool.

3. Grill the chicken breasts over medium heat for 7-8 minutes on each side, or until they reach an internal temperature of 165°F. Allow them to rest before slicing into strips.

4. In a large bowl, mix the chilled quinoa, sliced chicken, cherry tomatoes, cucumber, red onion, olives, and crumbled feta cheese.

5. Make the dressing by mixing the olive oil, lemon juice, salt, and pepper. Drizzle over the salad and toss to mix.

6. If wanted, serve the salad on a bed of mixed greens to boost nutrients and fiber.

COOKING TIPS

1. Marinate the chicken in a combination of olive oil, lemon juice, garlic, and herbs for at least 30 minutes before grilling to increase the taste.

2. Toast the quinoa in a pan for 2-3 minutes before cooking to bring out its nuttier taste.

Nutritional Values per Serving: Calories: Approximately 350-400 | Protein: 30g | Carbohydrates: 35g | Fats: 10g | Fiber: 6g

SERVING PORTION: THIS RECIPE SERVES 2 PEOPLE.

PREP TIME: 20 MINUTES (PLUS MARINATING TIME IF APPLICABLE)

COOK TIME: 30 MINUTES

NOTE: This meal was created with a prostate cancer diet in mind, emphasizing items that may help lower the risk of cancer and promote general health. It contains a wide range of colorful vegetables and fruits, nutritious grains such as quinoa, and healthy fats from olive oil and almonds, all of which are good for seniors with prostate cancer.

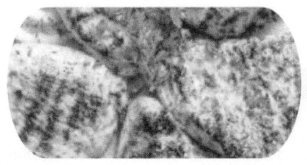
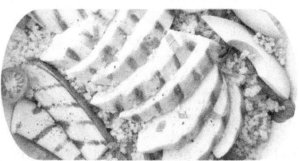

11. Quinoa and Black Bean Burrito Bowl

This Quinoa and Black Bean Burrito Bowl is a substantial, healthy dish ideal for seniors on a prostate cancer diet. It is high in proteins, fiber, and antioxidants, with an emphasis on components that promote a healthy lifestyle throughout cancer recovery.

INGREDIENTS:

- 1 cup of quinoa (rinsed)
- 2 cups of water or low-sodium vegetable broth
- 1 can (15 oz) of black beans (drained and rinsed)
- 1/2 cup of red onion (finely chopped)
- 1 clove garlic (minced)
- 1 tsp. of ground cumin
- 1/2 teaspoon of chili powder
- 1/4 cup of fresh cilantro (chopped)
- Juice of 1 lime
- 1 cup of cherry tomatoes (halved)
- 1 avocado (sliced)
- Salt and pepper to taste

INSTRUCTIONS:

1. In a medium saucepan, heat the quinoa and water until boiling. Reduce the heat to low, cover, and cook for 15-20 minutes until the quinoa is fluffy and the water has been absorbed.

2. While the quinoa is cooking, heat a nonstick pan over medium heat. Combine black beans, red onion, garlic, cumin, and chili powder. Cook for 5-7 minutes, until the onions are tender.

3. Remove the quinoa from the heat and cover it for 5 minutes. Fluff with a fork and add the lime juice and cilantro.

4. To assemble the bowls, divide the quinoa among serving plates. Top with black bean mixture, cherry tomatoes, and avocado slices. Season with salt and pepper, to taste.

COOKING TIPS:

1. Instead of using water, boil the quinoa in vegetable broth for extra flavor.

2. To avoid mushiness, let the cooked quinoa rest before fluffing.

3. Add the lime juice while the quinoa is still heated for better absorption and taste.

Nutritional Values per Serving: Calories: 340 | Protein: 14g | Fiber: 10g | Fat: 8g (mostly from avocado, which provides healthy fats) | Carbohydrates: 55g

SERVING PORTION: THIS RECIPE SERVES 4 PEOPLE.

PREP TIME: 10 MINUTES

COOK TIME: 20 MINUTES

NOTE: A prostate cancer-friendly diet should contain foods high in antioxidants and minimize intake of red meat and dairy items. This dish includes plant-based proteins and is rich in nutrients that are beneficial for general health and recovery.

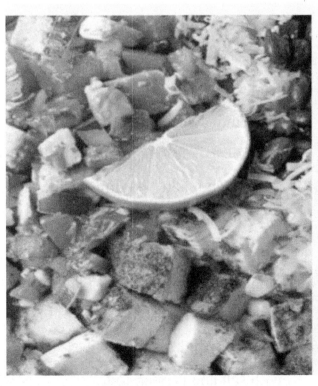
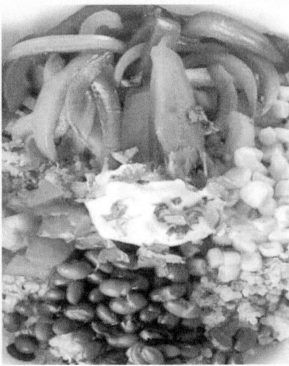

12. Roasted Vegetable and Hummus Wrap

This Roasted Vegetable and Hummus Wrap combines nutritious veggies and creamy hummus on a soft tortilla. It is ideal for adults seeking a nutritious meal that promotes a healthy prostate diet.

INGREDIENTS:

- 1 red bell pepper, sliced
- 1 yellow bell pepper, sliced
- 1 zucchini, sliced
- 1 yellow squash, sliced
- 1 red onion, sliced
- 2 tablespoons olive oil
- Salt and pepper, to taste
- 4 whole grain tortillas
- 1 cup of homemade or store-bought hummus
- 2 cups of fresh spinach leaves

INSTRUCTIONS:

1. Heat your oven to 400°F (200°C).

2. Transfer the cut veggies to a baking sheet. Drizzle with olive oil, then season with salt and pepper. Toss to coat evenly.

3. Roast the veggies in a preheated oven for 20-25 minutes, or until soft and slightly caramelized.

4. Heat the tortillas in the oven for a few minutes or in a pan over medium heat.

5. Spread a large amount of hummus over each tortilla.

6. Place a handful of spinach leaves on top of the hummus.

7. Spread the roasted veggies equally among the tortillas.

8. Roll the tortillas firmly, tucking the edges in.

9. Cut the wraps in half and serve immediately.

COOKING TIPS:

1. Roast the veggies with fresh herbs such as thyme or rosemary for extra flavor.

2. For a warm wrap, immediately reheat the assembled wraps in the oven before serving.

Nutritional Values Per Serving: Calories: Approximately 300-350 | Protein: 10g | Fiber: 6g | Fat: 15g (mostly from olive oil and hummus, which are healthy fats)

SERVING PORTION: THIS RECIPE MAKES 4 SERVINGS.

PREP TIME: 15 MINUTES TO SLICE VEGETABLES AND PREPARE INGREDIENTS.

COOK TIME: 20-25 MINUTES FOR ROASTING VEGETABLES.

NOTE: Enjoy this nourishing and tasty wrap, which is ideal for anybody looking for a healthy and enjoyable lunch, not just those on a prostate cancer diet.

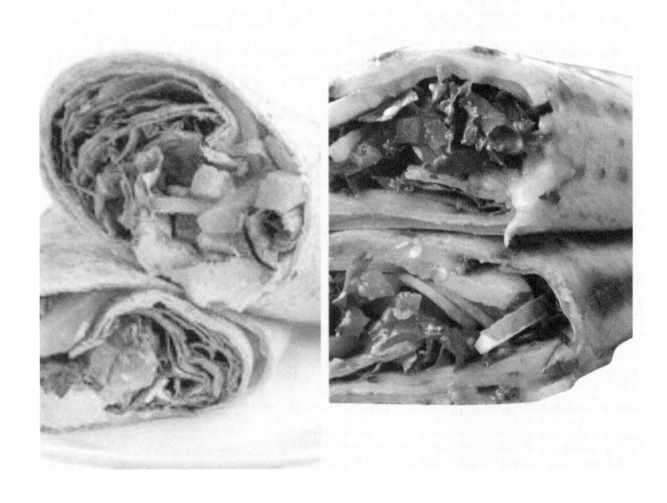

13. Asian Pan Seared Salmon Salad

This salad is a great way to include lean protein and a variety of veggies in your diet. Salmon is high in omega-3 fatty acids, which are good for your heart and joints. They may also help reduce inflammation related to prostate cancer.

INGREDIENTS:

- 4 salmon fillets (about 6 ounces each)
- Salt and pepper to taste
- 1 tablespoon of olive oil
- Mixed greens (such as romaine, spinach, and arugula)
- 1 red bell pepper, thinly sliced
- 1/2 cucumber, sliced
- 1 carrot, julienned
- 1/4 red onion, thinly sliced
- 1/4 cup of cilantro leaves
- 1 tablespoon of toasted sesame seeds

HONEY SESAME DRESSING:

- 2 tablespoons of soy sauce
- 1 tablespoon of sesame oil
- 1 tablespoon of honey
- 1 clove garlic, minced
- 1 teaspoon of grated fresh ginger

INSTRUCTIONS:

1. Season salmon fillets with salt and pepper.

2. Heat the olive oil in a pan over medium-high heat. Place the salmon fillets, skin side down, and sear for 4 minutes.

3. Flip the salmon and cook for a further 3 minutes, or until desired doneness.

4. In a large bowl, add the mixed greens, red bell pepper, cucumber, carrot, and red onion.

5. In a separate bowl, mix together the honey and sesame dressing ingredients.

6. Drizzle the salad with the dressing and toss to mix.

7. Top the salad with the grilled salmon and cilantro leaves, then sprinkle with toasted sesame seeds.

COOKING TIPS:

1. Before adding the salmon, heat the pan to ensure crisper skin.

2. Rest the salmon for a few minutes after cooking to ensure even juiciness.

Nutritional Values Per Serving: Calories: 370 | Fat: 20g | Carbohydrates: 12g | Protein: 34g | Fiber: 3g

SERVING PORTION: SERVES 4.

PREP TIME: 15 MINUTES.

COOK TIME: 10 MINUTES.

NOTE: This Asian Pan Seared Salmon Salad is a delicious and nutritious alternative for seniors on a prostate cancer diet. Fresh veggies and grilled fish, topped with a honey sesame sauce, make for a nutritious and enjoyable lunch.

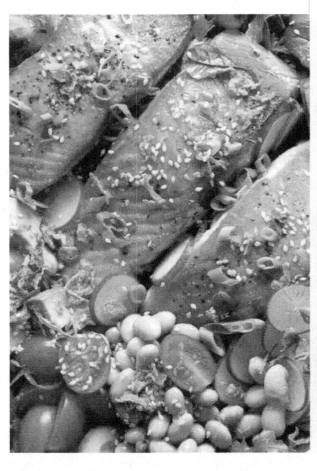
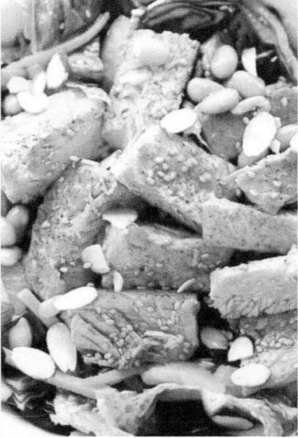

14. Pasta w/ Crispy Rosemary Chickpeas & Roasted Tomatoes

This pasta meal combines the heartiness of crispy rosemary chickpeas with the sweetness of roasted tomatoes, all served over your favorite pasta. It's a meal that's not only comforting but also full of prostate-healthy foods like tomatoes (high in lycopene) and chickpeas (high in plant-based protein and fiber).

INGREDIENTS:

- 8 oz of your preferred pasta (whole grain recommended)
- 1 can (15 oz) of chickpeas, drained and dried
- 2 cups of cherry tomatoes
- 2 sprigs fresh rosemary, leaves stripped and minced
- 3 tbsp. of olive oil, divided
- 2 cloves garlic, minced
- Salt and pepper, to taste
- Grated Parmesan cheese, for serving (optional)

INSTRUCTIONS:

1. Heat your oven to 400°F (200°C).

2. Season the cherry tomatoes with 1 tablespoon olive oil, salt, and pepper. Spread them out on a baking sheet and roast for 20 minutes, until blistered and tender.

3. Meanwhile, combine the chickpeas, rosemary, 1 tablespoon olive oil, salt, and pepper. Spread them out on a separate baking sheet and roast for 20 minutes, until crispy.

4. Cook the pasta according to package instructions until al dente. Drain and set aside.

5. In a big pan, heat the remaining olive oil over medium heat. Add the garlic and sauté until fragrant.

6. Combine the cooked pasta, roasted tomatoes, and crispy chickpeas in the pan. Toss to mix and heat well.

7. Serve hot, topped with grated Parmesan cheese if preferred.

COOKING TIPS:

1. Before roasting the tomatoes, add an addition of balsamic vinegar for added flavor.

2. To achieve crispness, properly dry the chickpeas before roasting.

3. Reserve some pasta water to add to the meal if it appears dry after mixing all of the ingredients.

Nutritional Values Per Serving: Calories: Approximately 350 kcal | Protein: 15 g | Fiber: 8 g | Fat: 10 g (healthy fats from olive oil) | Carbohydrates: 55 g

SERVING PORTION: THIS RECIPE SERVES 4 PEOPLE.

PREP TIME: 10 MINUTES

COOK TIME: 40 MINUTES (20 MINUTES FOR ROASTING TOMATOES AND CHICKPEAS, 20 MINUTES FOR PASTA COOKING AND COMBINING)

NOTE: This meal, like a prostate cancer diet for seniors, uses foods that promote a healthy diet. Including stewed tomatoes, which are rich in antioxidants, and choosing plant-based proteins like chickpeas over red meat can contribute to better living and may even reduce the chance of cancer growth.

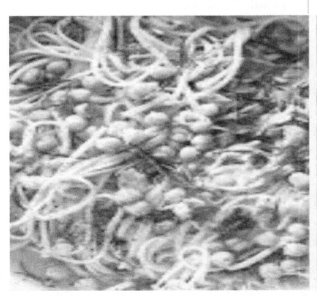 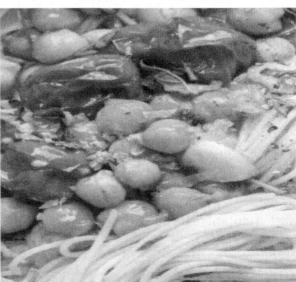

15. Herby Chicken Breasts

Herby Chicken Breasts are an easy and tasty way to get lean protein. This recipe infuses chicken with a variety of fragrant herbs, resulting in a meal that is both warm and nourishing. It is especially great for seniors on a prostate cancer diet since it is low in fat and high in protein.

INGREDIENTS:

- 4 boneless, skinless chicken breasts
- 2 tbsp. of olive oil
- 1 lemon, juice and zest
- 2 cloves garlic, minced
- 1 tsp. of dried oregano
- 1 tsp. of dried thyme
- 1 tsp. of dried parsley
- 1/2 tsp. of dried sage
- 1/2 tsp. of dried rosemary
- Salt and pepper, to taste

INSTRUCTIONS:

1. To make the marinade, mix olive oil, lemon juice, zest, garlic, and herbs in a bowl.

2. Season the chicken breasts with salt and pepper, then coat them in the marinade. Allow them to settle for at least 20 minutes, or overnight in the refrigerator for a richer flavor.

3. Heat your oven to 375°F (190°C).

4. Transfer the marinated chicken breasts to a baking tray and bake for 25-30 minutes, or until the internal temperature reaches 165°F (75°C).

5. Rest the chicken for 5 minutes before slicing.

1. Marinating the chicken for a longer time will enhance the taste.

2. Allowing the chicken to rest after baking promotes juiciness.

3. Serve with steamed veggies for a well-balanced meal.

Nutritional Values Per Serving: Calories: Approximately 220 kcal | Protein: 35 g | Fat: 9 g | Carbohydrates: 1 g | Fiber: 0.5 g | Sodium: 70 mg

SERVING PORTION: THIS RECIPE SERVES 4 PEOPLE.

PREP TIME: 10 MINUTES (PLUS MARINATING TIME)

COOK TIME: 25-30 MINUTES

NOTE: Cooked tomatoes and cruciferous vegetables, such as broccoli and cauliflower, are high in antioxidants and should be included in a prostate cancer diet. Lean proteins, such as chicken and plant-based proteins, are also suggested. This Herby Chicken Breast dish follows these standards, providing a nutritious and tasty option for seniors.

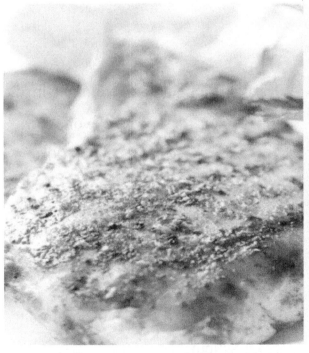
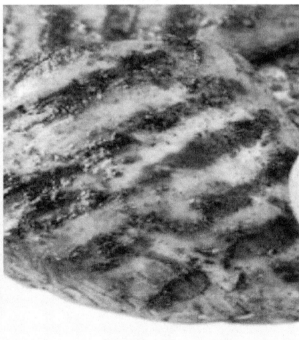

CHAPTER 5: DINNER DIET FOR PROSTATE HEALTH

1. Thyme-Lemon Marinated Chicken

Thyme-Lemon Marinated Chicken is a zesty and herbaceous recipe that adds a fresh edge to your meal. Lemon and thyme not only give the chicken an amazing taste, but they also have antioxidant and anti-inflammatory effects. This meal is ideal for seniors following a prostate cancer diet, as it promotes lean proteins and avoids processed meats.

INGREDIENTS:

- 4 boneless, skinless chicken breasts
- 1/4 cup of olive oil
- 1/4 cup of fresh lemon juice
- 4 garlic cloves, grated or minced
- 1 tablespoon of dried thyme
- 1 teaspoon of salt
- 1/2 teaspoon of ground black pepper

INSTRUCTIONS:

1. Combine olive oil, lemon juice, garlic, thyme, salt, and pepper in a large zip-top plastic bag to make the marinade.

2. Place the chicken breasts in the bag, close, and flip to coat evenly. Marinate in the refrigerator for 30 minutes to 2 hours.

3. Preheat the oven to 450 degrees Fahrenheit (230 degrees Celsius).

4. Arrange the chicken in a single layer in an oven-safe pan or baking dish. Pour any remaining marinade over the chicken.

5. Bake uncovered for 15 minutes, then flip the chicken skin side up and bake for a further 15 minutes, or until well done.

COOKING TIPS:

1. Avoid marinating the chicken for too long since the citrus can change the texture of the flesh.

2. Allow the chicken to rest for a few minutes after cooking to ensure tender and juicy flesh.

3. To increase the nutritional value of this dish, serve it with steamed vegetables or a fresh salad.

Nutritional Values Per Serving: Calories: Approximately 300 kcal | Protein: 26 g | Fat: 20 g (mostly from olive oil, which is a healthier fat option) | Carbohydrates: 3 g | Fiber: 0.5 g | Sodium: 600 mg

SERVING PORTION: THIS RECIPE SERVES 4 PEOPLE.

PREP TIME: 10 MINUTES (PLUS AT LEAST 30 MINUTES FOR MARINATING)

COOK TIME: 30 MINUTES

NOTE: A prostate cancer diet for seniors should include foods strong in antioxidants and low in saturated fats.

This Thyme-Lemon Marinated Chicken dish is an excellent choice since it utilizes olive oil instead of butter and emphasizes lean protein.

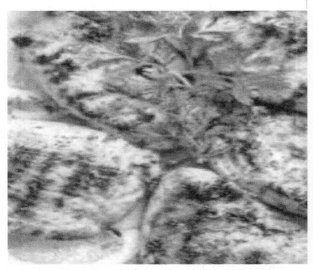 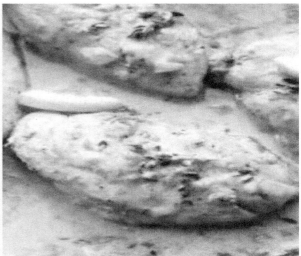

2. Ginger-Garlic Shrimp Stir Fry

Ginger-Garlic Shrimp Stir Fry is a colorful and nutritious dish that mixes the bold tastes of ginger and garlic with the delicious shrimp. It's a quick and easy meal that's ideal for seniors, with a decent combination of protein, vitamins, and antioxidants that are necessary for prostate cancer treatment.

INGREDIENTS:

- 1 pound (454 g) large shrimp, peeled and deveined
- 2 tablespoons of cornstarch
- Salt and pepper, to taste
- 1/3 cup (79 ml) of soy sauce
- 1/3 cup (113 g) of honey
- 2 cloves garlic, minced
- 2 tablespoons of finely minced fresh ginger
- Sesame seeds, for topping
- Green onions, for topping
- Vegetable oil for cooking

INSTRUCTIONS:

1. In a measuring cup, combine soy sauce, honey, minced garlic, and minced ginger to make the sauce.

2. In a large bowl, combine shrimp, cornstarch, salt, and pepper. Toss to coat evenly.

3. Heat a little amount of vegetable oil in a medium pan over medium-high heat. Once heated, add the shrimp and fry until they are crispy on both sides.

4. Remove the shrimp from the skillet and set them aside.

5. Keeping the heat on, add the sauce to the skillet and cook to a moderate simmer until thickened.

6. Once the sauce has thickened, add the shrimp and toss to coat.

7. Remove from heat and garnish with sesame seeds and green onions, if preferred.

8. Serve with white or brown rice.

COOKING TIPS:

1. Before frying, coat the shrimp well with cornstarch for a crunchy texture.

2. Cook the shrimp in batches if required to avoid overloading the pan.

3. Adjust the amount of ginger and garlic to your liking.

Nutritional Values Per Serving: Calories: Approximately 373 kcal | Protein: 56 g | Carbohydrates: 58 g | Sugar: 46 g

SERVING PORTION: THIS RECIPE SERVES 2 PEOPLE.

PREP TIME: 5 MINUTES

COOK TIME: 15 MINUTES

NOTE: Including this dish in a prostate cancer diet is beneficial since it is high in protein and contains ginger and garlic, both of which are anti-inflammatory.

A healthy diet should include a mix of vegetables and lean proteins while limiting red meat and processed items.

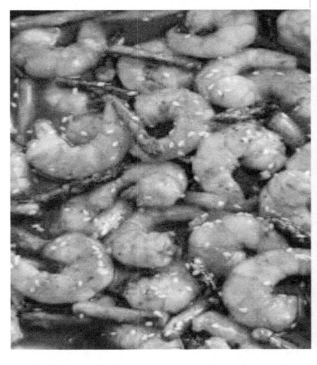
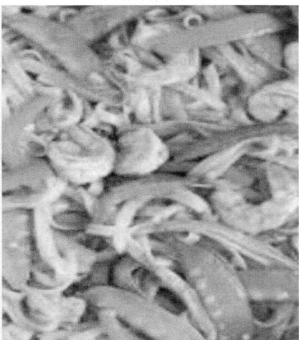

3. Spaghetti Squash with Turkey Bolognese

Spaghetti Squash with Turkey Bolognese is a satisfying and healthy low-carb alternative to classic pasta recipes. The turkey provides lean protein, and the spaghetti squash is an enjoyable and fiber-rich pasta substitute, making it great for seniors concerned about their prostate health.

INGREDIENTS:

- 1 large spaghetti squash
- 1 lb. of ground turkey (93% lean)
- 1 medium onion, finely chopped
- 2 cloves garlic, minced
- 1 carrot, diced
- 1 can (28 oz) of crushed tomatoes
- 1/4 cup of tomato paste
- 1/4 cup of fresh basil, chopped
- 1 tsp. of dried oregano
- Salt and pepper, to taste
- 2 tbsp. of olive oil
- Grated Parmesan cheese, for serving (optional)

INSTRUCTIONS:

1. Heat the oven to 400°F (200°C). Split the spaghetti squash lengthwise and remove the seeds. Place cut-side down on a baking sheet and roast for approximately 40 minutes, or until soft.

2. While the squash roasts, warm the olive oil in a large pan over medium heat. Add the onion and garlic and cook until transparent.

3. Place the ground turkey in the skillet and heat until browned.

4. Mix in the carrots, smashed tomatoes, tomato paste, basil, oregano, salt, and pepper. Simmer for 20 minutes, letting the flavors combine.

5. When the squash is finished, use a fork to scrape out the "spaghetti" threads.

6. Pour the turkey bolognese sauce over the spaghetti squash strands and, if preferred, sprinkle with grated Parmesan cheese.

COOKING TIPS:

1. Allow the bolognese sauce to boil for a further 10-15 minutes to add more flavor.

2. You may add a small amount of red wine to the sauce to give it depth.

3. Keep any leftovers in an airtight jar in the refrigerator for up to 3 days.

Nutritional Values Per Serving: Calories: Approximately 320 kcal | Protein: 27 g | Fat: 12 g | Carbohydrates: 28 g | Fiber: 6 g | Sodium: 300 mg

SERVING PORTION: THIS RECIPE SERVES 4 PEOPLE.

PREP TIME: 15 MINUTES

COOK TIME: 1 HOUR (INCLUDES ROASTING THE SQUASH AND SIMMERING THE SAUCE)

NOTE: This meal is consistent with a prostate cancer diet for seniors, focusing on veggies, lean meats, and healthy fats while reducing red meat and processed foods. The use of stewed tomatoes, which are high in lycopene, and lean turkey instead of red meat make this recipe a good option for those maintaining prostate health.

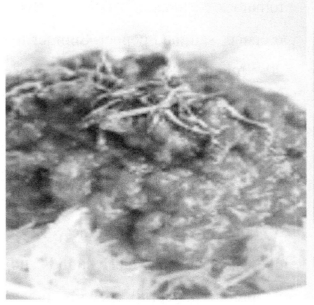
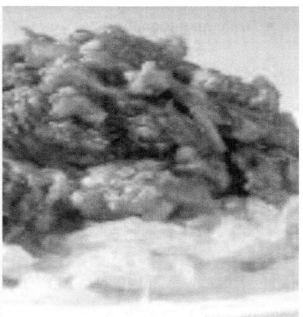

4. Grilled Vegetable and Chicken Kebabs

Grilled Vegetables and Chicken Kebabs are an ideal mix of lean protein and a variety of veggies, making them a nutritious and tasty complement to any meal. This meal is especially excellent for seniors on a prostate cancer diet since it has low-fat, high-antioxidant components.

INGREDIENTS:

- 4 boneless, skinless chicken breasts, cut into cubes
- 1 zucchini, sliced into rounds
- 1 yellow squash, sliced into rounds
- 1 red bell pepper, cut into chunks
- 1 green bell pepper, cut into chunks
- 1 red onion, cut into chunks
- Olive oil for brushing
- Salt and pepper, to taste
- Fresh herbs (like rosemary or thyme), finely chopped, for marinade

INSTRUCTIONS:

1. Heat your grill to medium-high.

2. In a bowl, combine olive oil, salt, pepper, and fresh herbs to make a marinate.

3. Toss the chicken and veggies in the marinade until evenly covered.

4. Thread the chicken and veggies on skewers, rotating between them.

5. Grill the kebabs for 10-15 minutes, flipping regularly, until the chicken is fully cooked and the veggies are soft yet crunchy.

COOKING TIPS:

1. Soak wooden skewers in water for at least 30 minutes before grilling to avoid scorching.

2. Cut the chicken and veggies into equal-sized pieces to promote uniform cooking.

3. Brush the kebabs with extra olive oil while grilling to keep them moist and delicious.

Nutritional Values Per Serving: Calories: Approximately 250 kcal | Protein: 26 g | Fat: 9 g | Carbohydrates: 15 g | Fiber: 3 g | Sodium: 200 mg

SERVING PORTION: THIS RECIPE MAKES 4 SERVINGS.

PREP TIME: 20 MINUTES (INCLUDING MARINATING TIME)

COOK TIME: 10-15 MINUTES

NOTE: A prostate cancer diet should contain a mix of vegetables and lean proteins while avoiding red meat and processed foods. This meal includes chicken as a lean protein source and a combination of colorful veggies, both of which are advised for this diet.

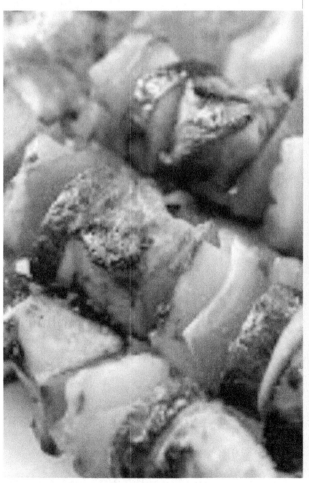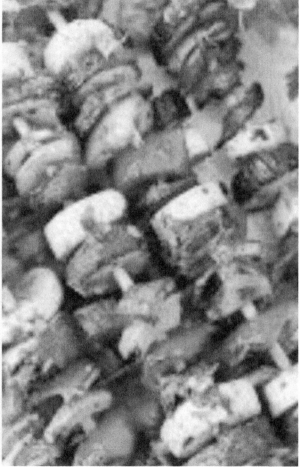

5. Zucchini Noodles with Pesto and Cherry Tomatoes

Zucchini Noodles with Pesto and Cherry Tomatoes are a colorful and refreshing dish that's ideal for a light lunch or dinner. It's a great low-carb alternative to regular pasta that's high in vitamins and antioxidants. Cherry tomatoes give a blast of flavor and a dose of lycopene, which is good for your prostate.

INGREDIENTS:

- 2 medium-sized zucchinis
- 1/2 cup of cherry tomatoes, cut in half
- 2 tablespoons of store-bought or homemade pesto
- 1 tablespoon of olive oil
- Salt and pepper, to taste
- Shaved Parmesan cheese, for garnish (optional)

INSTRUCTIONS:

1. Use a spiralizer or a vegetable peeler to make zucchini noodles (zoodles).

2. Heat 1 tablespoon of olive oil in a pan over medium heat.

3. Add the cherry tomatoes and cook for 1 minute.

4. Stir in the pesto and zucchini noodles.

5. Season with salt and pepper and stir thoroughly.

6. Cook for a further 2 minutes, or until the zoodles are tender.

7. Remove from the heat and garnish with shaved Parmesan cheese, if preferred.

8. Serve immediately and enjoy!

COOKING TIPS:

1. Avoid overcooking the zoodles to keep them from getting mushy.

2. If you like a crunchier texture, shorten the cooking time for the zoodles.

3. For more protein, try topping with grilled chicken or shrimp.

Nutritional Values Per Serving: Calories: Approximately 150 kcal | Protein: 4 g | Fat: 12 g (healthy fats from olive oil and pesto) | Carbohydrates: 8 g | Fiber: 2 g | Sodium: 250 mg

SERVING PORTION: THIS RECIPE SERVES 2 PEOPLE.

PREP TIME: 10 MINUTES

COOK TIME: 5 MINUTES

NOTE: This dish complies with a prostate cancer diet for seniors, emphasizing veggies and healthy fats while avoiding processed foods and red meat.

The use of zucchini as a noodle substitute is an excellent approach to improve vegetable consumption, while the olive oil and pesto give healthy fats that are necessary for a well-balanced diet.

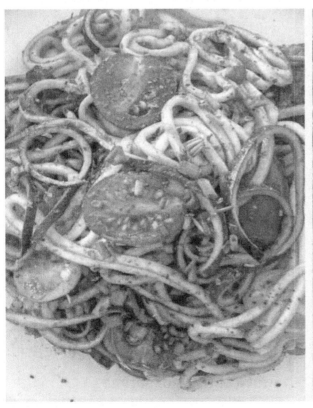 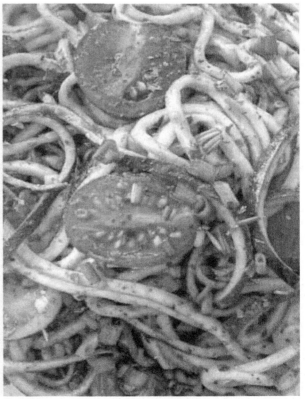

6. Grilled Tofu and Vegetable Skewers

Grilled Tofu and Vegetable Skewers are a delicious way to enjoy a variety of veggies while also getting some plant-based nutrition from tofu. This meal is perfect for seniors on a prostate cancer diet since it is high in nutrients, low in fat, and does not include red or processed meats.

INGREDIENTS:

- 1 block (14 oz) of extra-firm tofu, drained and pressed
- 1 zucchini, cut into 1/2-inch slices
- 1 yellow squash, cut into 1/2-inch slices
- 1 red onion, cut into chunks
- 1 red bell pepper, cut into chunks
- 2/3 cup of chopped Italian parsley
- 2 tsp. of dried oregano
- 2 tbsp. of finely chopped shallot
- 2 tsp. of minced garlic
- 2 tsp. of honey
- 6 tbsp. of red wine vinegar
- 2/3 cup of extra-virgin olive oil
- Salt and freshly ground black pepper, to taste
- 1/2 cup of toasted pine nuts
- Warm naan or pita, for serving

INSTRUCTIONS:

1. Cut the tofu into 12 equal pieces and lay on a dish lined with paper towels to dry.

2. Place the tofu, zucchini, yellow squash, red onion, and bell pepper on skewers.

3. In a bowl, mix together the parsley, oregano, shallots, garlic, honey,

vinegar, oil, salt, and pepper to make the marinade.

4. Set aside 2/3 cup of the marinade for serving, and brush the remainder onto the skewers.

5. Preheat the grill to medium-high heat, then gently oil the grates.

6. Grill the skewers, turning often, until the tofu is grill-marked and the veggies are cooked through about 16-20 minutes.

7. Serve the skewers with the remaining marinade and warm naan or pita.

COOKING TIPS:

1. To eliminate extra moisture and improve the texture of the tofu, press it.

2. Soak wooden skewers in water for 30 minutes to avoid burning.

3. Grill the skewers covered to achieve consistent cooking and prevent drying.

Nutritional Values Per Serving: Calories: Approximately 450 kcal | Protein: 19 g | Fat: 35 g | Carbohydrates: 15 g | Fiber: 4 g | Sodium: 200 mg

SERVING PORTION: THIS RECIPE SERVES 4 PEOPLE.

PREP TIME: 15 MINUTES (EXCLUDING MARINATING TIME)

COOK TIME: 20 MINUTES

NOTE:A prostate cancer diet should include plant-based proteins and a variety of vegetables while limiting saturated fats and avoiding processed meats. Tofu is used as a healthy protein source in this meal, along with a variety of bright veggies, which aligns with prostate health dietary guidelines.

7. Spinach and Mushroom Stuffed Chicken Breast

Spinach & Mushroom Stuffed Chicken Breast mixes delicate chicken, garlicky mushrooms, spinach, and a layer of melted cheese. It's a simple yet remarkable recipe that turns chicken breast into a delicious dinner.

INGREDIENTS:

- 4 boneless, skinless chicken breasts
- 1 tbsp. of olive oil
- Salt and pepper, to taste
- 1 cup of baby spinach, chopped
- 1 cup of mushrooms, sliced
- 2 cloves garlic, minced
- 1/2 cup of shredded mozzarella cheese (or any melting cheese of your choice)
- Fresh thyme or rosemary, for garnish (optional)

INSTRUCTIONS:

1. Heat your oven to 375°F (190°C).

2. In a pan, heat the olive oil over medium heat. Add the minced garlic and cook until fragrant.

3. Cook the sliced mushrooms until they release moisture and turn golden brown.

4. Stir in the chopped spinach and simmer until wilted. Season with salt and pepper.

5. Butterfly the chicken breasts by creating a pocket in each one, taking care not to cut all the way through.

6. Stuff each chicken breast with mushroom-spinach mixture and grated mozzarella cheese.

7. Use toothpicks to seal the pockets and hold the contents in place.

8. Season the outsides of the chicken breasts with salt and pepper.

9. Cook in a skillet over medium-high heat. Add a sprinkle of olive oil.

10. Cook the filled chicken breasts for about 2 minutes per side until golden brown.

11. Place the pan in the heated oven for 15-20 minutes, or until the chicken is cooked through.

12. Remove the toothpicks before serving.

13. Optional: garnish with fresh thyme or rosemary.

COOKING TIPS:

1. For tasty bits, use a substantial amount of filling.

2. Using toothpicks, partly close the pockets, allowing some cheese to leak out during baking.

3. Serve over steamed veggies or a simple salad.

Nutritional Values Per Serving: Calories: Approximately 300 kcal | Protein: 40 g | Fat: 10 g | Carbohydrates: 5 g | Fiber: 1 g | Sodium: 400 mg

SERVING PORTION: THIS RECIPE SERVES 4 PEOPLE.

PREP TIME: 20 MINUTES

COOK TIME: 20 MINUTES (INCLUDING SEARING AND BAKING)

NOTE: This Spinach and Mushroom Stuffed Chicken Breast is a delicious complement to any dinner table. It's high in protein and minerals, making it a great option for seniors on a prostate cancer diet.

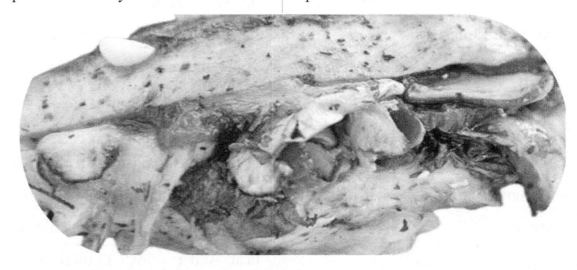

9. Sweet and Spicy Grilled Shrimp

Sweet & Spicy Grilled Shrimp is a delicious meal that combines shrimp's essential sweetness with a tangy, spicy sauce. It's a simple but delicious way to eat seafood, and it's particularly suitable for seniors looking for tasty foods that conform to a prostate cancer diet.

INGREDIENTS:

- 6 bamboo skewers, soaked in water for 20 minutes
- 1/2 cup of chile-garlic sauce
- 1/2 cup of honey
- 1 pound of medium shrimp, peeled and deveined

INSTRUCTIONS:

1. Preheat your grill to medium heat and gently oil the grilles.

2. Combine chile-garlic sauce and honey in a small bowl.

3. Thread the shrimp onto the moistened bamboo skewers, piercing both the head and tail ends.

4. Cook the skewers on the prepared grill, turning often and basting with the sauce mixture, until the shrimp are firm and pink on both sides, about 10 minutes.

COOKING TIPS:

1. Soak the bamboo skewers to keep them from burning on the grill.

2. To improve the taste, baste the shrimp with the sauce mixture while they cook.

3. To complete the food, serve with a side of steamed vegetables or a fresh salad.

Nutritional Values Per Serving: Calories: Approximately 231 kcal | Fat: 1g | Carbohydrates: 38g | Protein: 19g

SERVING PORTION: THIS RECIPE SERVES 4 PEOPLE.

PREP TIME: 10 MINUTES

COOK TIME: 10 MINUTES

NOTE: For seniors on a prostate cancer diet, it is important to include meals powerful in protein and low in saturated fat. Shrimp is a wonderful source of lean protein, and when combined with a range of vegetables, it may contribute to a balanced and healthy diet.

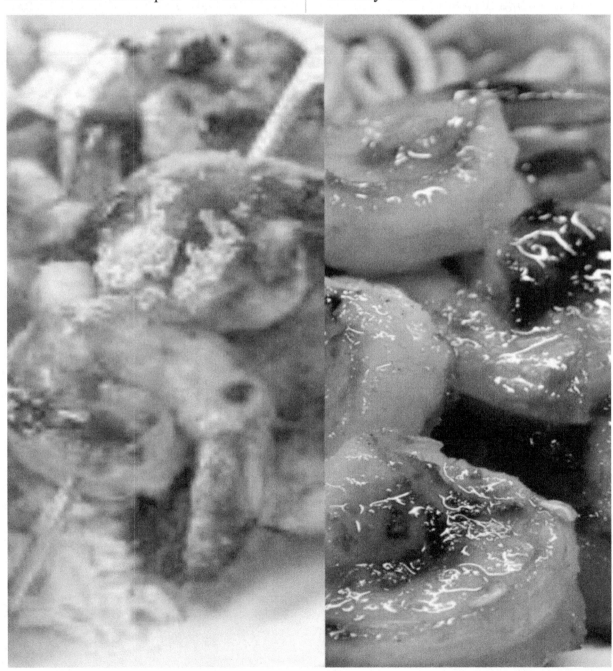

10. Maple Glazed Ginger Brussels Sprouts

Maple Glazed Ginger Brussels Sprouts add a sweet and spicy twist to traditional roasted Brussels sprouts. The natural sweetness of maple syrup matches the heat of the ginger, resulting in a side dish that is not only tasty but also high in cancer-fighting elements suitable for a prostate cancer diet.

INGREDIENTS:

- 2.5 pounds of Brussels sprouts
- 3 teaspoons of olive oil
- 1/2 teaspoon of salt
- 1/4 teaspoon of black pepper
- 1 clove garlic, grated
- 1 teaspoon of grated ginger
- 3 tablespoons of pure maple syrup
- 1 tablespoon of sesame oil
- 2 teaspoons of tamari or soy sauce
- Optional garnishes: toasted sesame seeds, red pepper flakes

INSTRUCTIONS:

1. Heat the oven to 400°F (200°C).

2. Wash the Brussels sprouts, remove the stem ends, and cut in half.

3. On a baking sheet, sprinkle the Brussels sprouts with olive oil, salt, and pepper.

4. Roast Brussels sprouts for 25 minutes.

5. While the Brussels sprouts roast, combine the maple syrup, sesame oil, tamari, garlic, and ginger in a small bowl.

6. Remove the Brussels sprouts from the oven and pour the sauce mixture over them, tossing until well blended.

7. Put them back in the oven for another 10 minutes.

8. If preferred, garnish with toasted sesame seeds and red pepper flakes right before serving.

COOKING TIPS:

1. Ensure the Brussels sprouts are in a single layer on the baking sheet for even roasting.

2. For a deeper flavor, you can add a splash of balsamic vinegar to the glaze.

3. The optional garnishes of sesame seeds and red pepper flakes add texture and a spicy kick.

Nutritional Values Per Serving: Calories: Approximately 150 kcal | Protein: 5 g | Fat: 7 g | Carbohydrates: 20 g | Fiber: 4 g | Sodium: 200 mg

SERVING PORTION: THIS RECIPE SERVES 4-6 PEOPLE.

PREP TIME: 15 MINUTES

COOK TIME: 35 MINUTES

NOTE: Brussels sprouts are a great option for seniors on a prostate cancer diet because they contain high levels of antioxidants and other cancer-fighting compounds. The inclusion of ginger and garlic not only improves the flavor but also gives further anti-inflammatory benefits.

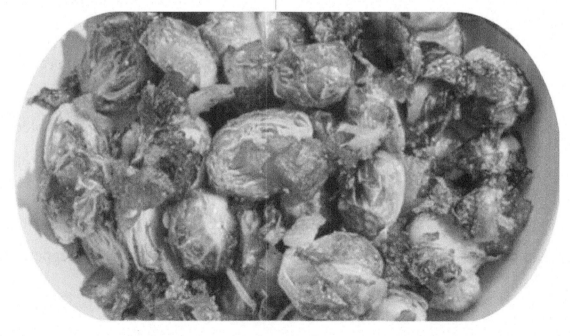

11. Vegetarian Enchilada Pasta

Vegetarian Enchilada Pasta is a filling and spicy dish that mixes the satisfying textures of pasta with the rich, strong flavors of enchilada sauce. It's high in nutrients from a range of vegetables and legumes, making it a great option for seniors trying to maintain a balanced diet post prostate cancer treatment.

INGREDIENTS:

- 8 oz. of Chickpea Pasta (or any other high-protein, gluten-free pasta)
- 2.5 cups of red enchilada sauce (homemade or store-bought)
- 1/2-1 cup of refried beans
- 1 cup of crushed tomatoes
- 2 cups of vegetable broth
- 1 cup of frozen corn (canned works too!)
- 1 cup of black beans, drained and rinsed
- 1 cup of pinto beans, drained and rinsed
- 1 cup of chickpeas, drained and rinsed
- 1 cup of lentils, cooked
- Optional toppings: avocado, cilantro, lime wedges

INSTRUCTIONS:

1. Cook the pasta according to package instructions until al dente, then drain and put aside.

2. In a large saucepan, mix the enchilada sauce, refried beans, crushed tomatoes, and vegetable broth. Stir until well combined.

3. Combine the cooked pasta, maize, black beans, pinto beans, chickpeas, and lentils in the saucepan.

4. Bring the mixture to a boil, then decrease the heat and simmer for 10 minutes, stirring regularly.

5. Serve hot, with optional toppings such as sliced avocado, chopped cilantro, and a squeeze of lime.

COOKING TIPS:

1. To make a smoother sauce, combine the refried beans and enchilada sauce before adding to the saucepan.

2. If necessary, add extra vegetable broth to the sauce to adjust its thickness.

3. The pasta will continue to absorb the sauce after standing, so add a bit more liquid if you want it saucier.

Nutritional Values Per Serving: Calories: Approximately 350 kcal | Protein: 18 g | Fat: 3 g | Carbohydrates: 65 g | Fiber: 15 g | Sodium: 700 mg

SERVING PORTION: THIS RECIPE SERVES 4 PEOPLE.

PREP TIME: 15 MINUTES

COOK TIME: 20 MINUTES

NOTE: This Vegetarian Enchilada Pasta is a great addition to a prostate cancer diet for seniors since it is strong in plant-based proteins and low in saturated fats. It contains a range of vegetables and legumes, which are essential components of a healthy diet that promotes recovery and general health.

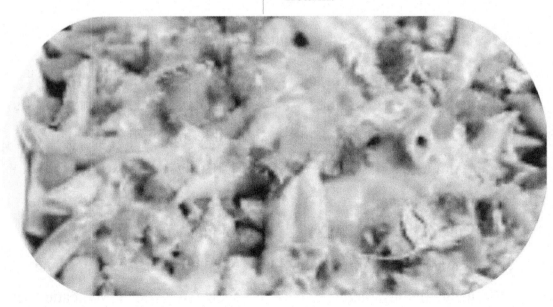

12. Turkey-Broccoli Stir-Fry

A prostate cancer diet for seniors should include lean proteins, fruits, vegetables, and whole grains while avoiding processed meals and red meats. This Turkey-Broccoli Stir-Fry dish follows those requirements, using lean turkey and broccoli, which is known for its cancer-fighting properties.

INGREDIENTS:

- 1 lb. of ground turkey
- 4 cups of broccoli florets
- 1 tablespoon of olive oil
- 2 cloves garlic, minced
- 1 red bell pepper, sliced
- 1/4 cup of low-sodium soy sauce
- 1 tablespoon of cornstarch
- 1/2 cup of chicken broth
- 1 tablespoon of honey
- 1 teaspoon of fresh ginger, grated
- Salt and pepper to taste

INSTRUCTIONS:

1. Heat the olive oil in a large pan over medium-high heat.

2. Cook the ground turkey until browned. Season with salt and pepper.

3. Remove the turkey from the skillet and put it aside.

4. In the same pan, sauté the garlic and red bell pepper for about 2 minutes, using additional oil as required.

5. Add the broccoli florets and cook until brilliant green and tender-crisp.

6. In a small bowl, combine the soy sauce, cornstarch, chicken broth, honey, and ginger.

7. Return the turkey to the pan with the veggies and pour the sauce mixture on top.

8. Cook for a few more minutes, or until the sauce thickens and everything is thoroughly covered.

9. Taste and adjust spice as needed.

COOKING TIPS:

1. Cut the broccoli into similar-sized florets to ensure consistent cooking.

2. If you want a thicker sauce, add the cornstarch slightly.

3. Serve it with brown rice or quinoa for a balanced meal.

Nutritional Values Per Serving: Calories: Approximately 250 kcal | Protein: 27 g | Fat: 11 g | Carbohydrates: 15 g | Fiber: 3 g | Sodium: 300 mg

SERVING PORTION: THIS RECIPE SERVES 4 PEOPLE.

PREP TIME: 10 MINUTES

COOK TIME: 20 MINUTES

NOTE: This Turkey-Broccoli Stir-Fry is a nutritious and delicious meal that fits well into a prostate cancer diet for seniors, offering critical nutrients without sacrificing flavor.

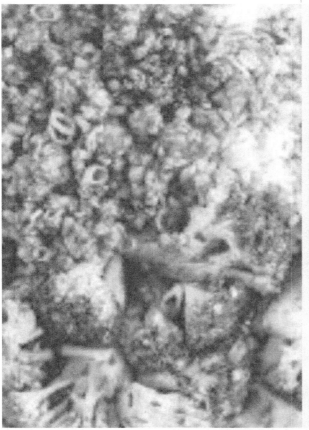
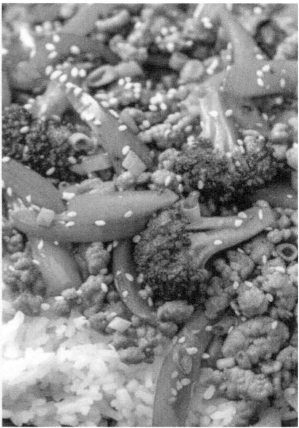

13. Sautéed Polenta with Butter Beans

Seniors recovering from prostate cancer should eat a diet rich in vegetables, fruits, complete grains, and lean meats. This Sautéed Polenta with Butter Beans dish is ideal since it contains high-fiber beans as well as polenta, a whole grain. It is also seasoned with beneficial spices and cooked in olive oil, which contains healthy fats.

INGREDIENTS:

- 4 teaspoons of extra-virgin olive oil, divided
- 1 16-ounce tube of plain polenta, cut into 1/2-inch cubes
- 1 clove garlic, minced
- 1 small onion, halved and thinly sliced
- 1 red bell pepper, diced
- 1/2 teaspoon of smoked paprika, plus more for garnish
- 1 15-ounce can of butter beans, rinsed
- 4 cups packed of baby spinach
- 3/4 cup of vegetable broth
- 1/2 cup of shredded Manchego or Monterey Jack cheese
- 2 teaspoons of sherry vinegar

INSTRUCTIONS:

1. Heat 2 teaspoons of oil in a large nonstick pan over medium-high heat.

2. Cook, stirring frequently, until the polenta cubes begin to brown, about 8 to 10 minutes. Transfer to a plate.

3. Reduce the heat to medium, then add the remaining oil and garlic to the pan. Cook for approximately 30 seconds, or until fragrant.

4. Cook until the onion and bell pepper are soft, about 3 to 5 minutes.

5. Sprinkle it with paprika and heat for an additional 30 seconds.

6. Add the beans, spinach, and stock; cook until the beans are cooked

through and the spinach has wilted, about 2 to 3 minutes.

7. Remove from heat and toss in cheese and vinegar.

8. Spread the vegetable and bean mixture over the sautéed polenta. If desired, sprinkle with extra paprika.

COOKING TIPS:

1. To get a crispy exterior, don't stir the polenta too much when sautéing.

2. Smoked paprika enhances the flavor, although sweet paprika can be used instead if preferred.

3. Red wine vinegar can be used instead of sherry vinegar to get a similar tart flavor.

Nutritional Values Per Serving: Calories: Approximately 221 kcal | Fat: 9g | Carbohydrates: 28g | Protein: 10g

SERVING PORTION: THIS RECIPE SERVES 4 PEOPLE, WITH 1 1/2 CUPS PER SERVING.

PREP TIME: 10 MINUTES

COOK TIME: 25 MINUTES

NOTE: This Sautéed Polenta with Butter Beans dish is a reliable and fulfilling meal that's consistent with the nutritional demands of seniors following a prostate cancer diet.

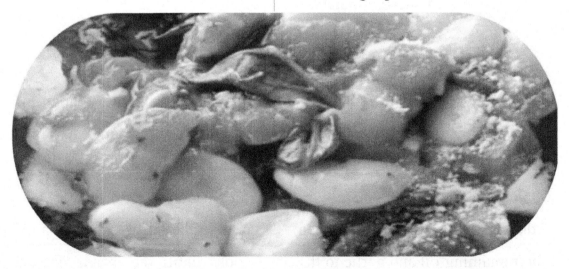

14. Parmesan Mushroom Casserole

A prostate cancer diet for seniors should include foods high in nutrition, fiber, and antioxidants but low in saturated fats. Mushrooms are a great option since they are low in calories, high in selenium, and have possible anti-cancer benefits. Parmesan provides a tasty touch of calcium and protein, making this meal a nutritious addition to a senior's diet.

INGREDIENTS:

- 1/4 cup of extra-virgin olive oil, plus 1 tablespoon, divided
- 1 cup of chopped onion
- 3 cloves of garlic, minced
- 2 pounds of baby bella mushrooms, sliced
- 3 tablespoons of all-purpose flour
- 3/4 teaspoon of salt
- 1/2 teaspoon of ground pepper
- 1/2 cup of sour cream
- 1/4 cup of Parmesan cheese, plus 1 tablespoon, divided
- 1/4 cup of chopped fresh parsley, plus 1 tablespoon, divided
- 1 tablespoon of lemon juice
- 1/4 cup of panko breadcrumbs

INSTRUCTIONS:

1. Heat your oven to 350°F (175°C). Coat an 8-inch square baking dish with cooking spray.

2. Heat 1/4 cup of oil in a large pan over medium heat. Cook for 3 minutes, or until the onion is tender and browning. Cook for 1 minute with the garlic.

3. Add the mushrooms in stages, stirring and allowing them to cook down before adding each handful until they're no longer opaque but still have some liquid in the pan.

4. Sprinkle flour, salt, and pepper over the veggies and cook, stirring, until thickened, about 1 to 2 minutes.

5. Remove from heat and mix in the sour cream, 1/4 cup Parmesan, 1/4 cup parsley, and lemon juice. Transfer to the prepared baking dish.

6. In a separate bowl, combine the panko, remaining 1 tablespoon oil, Parmesan, and parsley; stir well. Sprinkle the topping evenly over the mushroom mixture.

7. Bake for 20 to 25 minutes, or until the mixture bubbles and the breadcrumbs are gently toasted.

COOKING TIPS:

1. For a gluten-free version, substitute gluten-free flour and breadcrumbs.

2. To boost the umami taste, add a dash of soy sauce or Worcestershire sauce to the mushroom combination.

3. For a creamier texture, combine some of the cooked mushroom mixture before adding the sour cream and Parmesan.

Nutritional Values Per Serving: Calories: Approximately 229 kcal | Protein: 8g | Carbohydrates: 15g | Fiber: 2g | Sugars: 5g | Fat: 17g | Cholesterol: 13mg | Sodium: 387 mg | Potassium: 580mg

SERVING PORTION: THIS RECIPE SERVES 6 PEOPLE, WITH A SERVING SIZE OF ¾ CUP PER PERSON.

PREP TIME: 15 MINUTES

COOK TIME: 45 MINUTES (INCLUDING BAKING TIME)

NOTE: This Parmesan Mushroom Casserole is a delicious addition to a prostate cancer diet for seniors, providing a nutritious and delicious meal that is simple to make and enjoy.

15. Balsamic Chicken With Pears

A prostate cancer diet for seniors should focus on whole foods, lean meats, and a variety of fruits and vegetables. This Balsamic Chicken with Pears dish mixes pears' natural sweetness with tart balsamic vinegar, resulting in a delicious taste profile that is both gratifying and nutritious.

INGREDIENTS:

- 4 boneless, skinless chicken breast halves (about 6 ounces each)
- 3/4 teaspoon of salt
- 1/2 teaspoon of pepper
- 1 tablespoon of canola oil
- 1 cup of reduced-sodium chicken broth
- 3 tablespoons of white balsamic vinegar
- 1/2 teaspoon of minced fresh rosemary
- 2 teaspoons of cornstarch
- 1-1/2 teaspoons of sugar
- 2 medium unpeeled pears, each cut into 8 wedges
- 1/3 cup of dried cherries or dried cranberries

INSTRUCTIONS:

1. Season the chicken breasts with salt and pepper.

2. In a large nonstick skillet, heat the oil over medium-high heat. Add the chicken and cook for 8–10 minutes, or until a thermometer reads 165°F. Remove the chicken from the skillet.

3. In the meantime, mix the following five ingredients (chicken broth, white balsamic vinegar, minced rosemary, cornstarch, and sugar) until smooth. Pour the mixture into the skillet, then add the pears and dried cherries.

4. Bring the mixture to a boil over medium-high heat, then lower it to a

simmer and cover for 5 minutes, or until the pears are soft.

5. Return the chicken to the skillet and cook, uncovered, for 3–5 minutes.

6. If preferred, sprinkle with more minced rosemary.

7. Serve hot with rice or healthy grains.

COOKING TIPS:

1. Ripe pears provide the greatest flavor.

2. To adjust the sweetness, add more or less sugar to the sauce.

Nutritional Values Per Serving: Calories: 335 | Fat: 8g | Carbohydrates: 30g | Protein: 36g | Fiber: 3g

SERVING PORTION: THIS RECIPE SERVES 4 PEOPLE.

PREP TIME: 20 MINUTES

COOK TIME: 20 MINUTES

NOTE: This Balsamic Chicken with Pears is a delightful twist on the typical chicken-fruit-balsamic combination.

The addition of tomatoes and fresh basil adds depth and flavor.

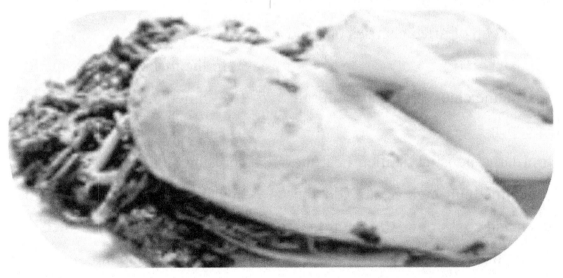

CHAPTER 6: PROSTATE-FRIENDLY SNACKS AND DESSERTS DIET

1. Coconut and Date Energy Bites

These energy bites are a nutritious, sweet treat ideal for seniors on a prostate cancer diet. They are produced with natural ingredients such as dates and coconut, which are high in fiber and healthy fats.

INGREDIENTS:

- 8 Medjool dates, pitted
- 1 cup of old-fashioned rolled oats
- 1/2 cup of unsweetened shredded coconut
- 2 tbsp. of raw honey
- 1 tbsp. of coconut oil, room temperature
- 1/8 tsp. of salt

INSTRUCTIONS:

1. Place the pitted dates in a food processor and pulse until broken down into smaller bits.

2. Add the oats, coconut, honey, oil, and salt and pulse until the mixture crumbles and is thoroughly combined.

3. Form the mixture into bite-sized balls and refrigerate in an airtight container until hard.

PREP TIPS:

1. To keep the final texture of the energy balls, do not over-process the mixture.

2. If the mixture is too dry, add more water to make it cling together.

Nutritional Values Per Serving: Calories: Approximately 100 kcal | Protein: 2 g | Fat: 4 g | Carbohydrates: 16 g | Fiber: 2 g

SERVING PORTION: MAKES 10 ENERGY BALLS.

PREP TIME: 10 MINUTES

2. Grilled Pineapple with Honey and Pistachios

Grilled pineapple with honey and pistachios is a sweet and savory dish that is simple to make and works well with a prostate cancer diet. Pineapple is high in vitamins and honey is a natural sweetener, so this is a healthy dessert option.

INGREDIENTS:

- 1 whole pineapple, peeled, cored, and cut into rings
- 1/4 cup of honey
- 1/2 cup of pistachios, chopped
- A pinch of cinnamon (optional)

INSTRUCTIONS:

1. Preheat the grill to medium.

2. In a small bowl, combine the honey and cinnamon.

3. Grill pineapple rings for 2-3 minutes on each side, or until heated through and with grill marks.

4. Drizzle the honey mixture over the grilled pineapple and garnish with chopped pistachios.

COOKING TIPS:

1. Allow the pineapple to marinade in the honey mixture before grilling for added flavor.

2. Avoid overcooking the pineapple to keep it juicy.

Nutritional Values Per Serving: Calories: Approximately 150 kcal | Protein: 1 g | Fat: 3 g | Carbohydrates: 30 g | Fiber: 2 g

SERVING PORTION: SERVES 4 PEOPLE.

PREP TIME: 10 MINUTES

COOK TIME: 6 MINUTES

3. Dark Chocolate and Almond Clusters

Dark chocolate contains antioxidants, and almonds are high in healthful fats and vitamin E, making these clusters a great snack for seniors on a prostate cancer diet.

INGREDIENTS:

- 1 cup of dark chocolate chips
- 1/2 cup of lightly salted almonds
- A sprinkle of kosher salt (optional)

INSTRUCTIONS:

1. Microwave the chocolate for 30-second intervals until completely melted.

2. Stir the almonds into the melted chocolate until covered.

3. Arrange the clusters in 1 tablespoon mounds on a silicone baking sheet.

4. Add salt if required.

PREP TIPS:

1. Use high-quality dark chocolate to improve both flavor and health benefits.

2. To add extra crunch, gently toast the almonds before mixing them into the chocolate.

Nutritional Values Per Serving: Calories: Approximately 150 kcal | Protein: 3 g | Fat: 11 g | Carbohydrates: 12 g | Fiber: 2 g

SERVING PORTION: THIS RECIPE MAKES ABOUT 10 CLUSTERS.

PREP TIME: 5 MINUTES

COOK TIME: 5 MINUTES (FOR MELTING CHOCOLATE)

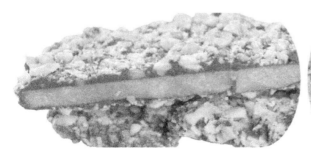
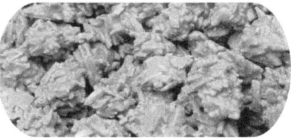

4. Baked Apples with Cinnamon and Walnuts

Baked apples are a delicious and warm dish rich in fiber and natural sugars. Cinnamon can help balance blood sugar levels, which is useful for seniors managing their diet following prostate cancer.

INGREDIENTS:

- 4 large apples
- 1/4 cup of maple syrup
- 1/2 cup of chopped walnuts
- 1 teaspoon of vanilla extract
- 1 teaspoon of cinnamon

INSTRUCTIONS:

1. Heat the oven to 350°F (175°C).

2. In a medium bowl, combine maple syrup, chopped walnuts, vanilla, and cinnamon.

3. Core four full apples, keeping their bottoms intact.

4. Fill the cored apples with walnut filling.

5. Bake for twenty minutes. Bake for an extra 10 minutes to make the apples softer.

COOKING TIPS:

1. Select firm apples, such as Gala or Honeycrisp, that will maintain their form when baked.

2. Serve warm, with a dollop of Greek yogurt for extra protein.

Nutritional Values Per Serving: Calories: Approximately 200 kcal | Protein: 2 g | Fat: 7 g | Carbohydrates: 35 g | Fiber: 5 g

SERVING PORTION: THIS RECIPE SERVES 4 PEOPLE.

PREP TIME: 10 MINUTES

COOK TIME: 20-30 MINUTES

5. Strawberry-Almond Cream Tart

This dessert is a delicious treat made with strawberries and almonds, both of which are good for the prostate. Strawberries are abundant in antioxidants, and almonds include nutritious fats and vitamin E.

INGREDIENTS:

- 36 honey graham crackers (about 9 sheets)
- 2 tablespoons of sugar
- 2 tablespoons of butter, melted
- 4 teaspoons of water
- 2/3 cup of light cream cheese
- 1/4 cup of sugar
- 1/2 teaspoon of vanilla extract
- 1/4 teaspoon of almond extract
- 6 cups of small, fresh strawberries
- 2/3 cup of sugar
- 1 tablespoon of cornstarch
- 1 tablespoon of fresh lemon juice
- 2 tablespoons of sliced almonds, toasted

INSTRUCTIONS:

1. Heat the oven to 350°F.

2. Process crackers until crumbs, then add sugar, butter, and water. Press into a tart pan.

3. Bake the crust for 10 minutes. Cool.

4. Combine cream cheese, sugar, and extracts; spread over the crust.

5. Puree 2 cups of strawberries and boil with sugar, cornstarch, and lemon juice until thickened.

6. Toss the remaining strawberries in the glaze and place them on the filling.

7. Allow it to chill for 3 hours.

COOKING TIPS:

1. To get a flakier texture, ensure that the crust components are chilled.

2. To keep the filling creamy, avoid overmixing.

Nutritional Values Per Serving: Calories: 289 | Fat: 8.9g | Carbohydrates: 48.7g |
Protein: 4.5g | Fiber: 3g

SERVING PORTION: SERVES 10.

PREP TIME: 20 MINUTES.

COOK TIME: 10 MINUTES.

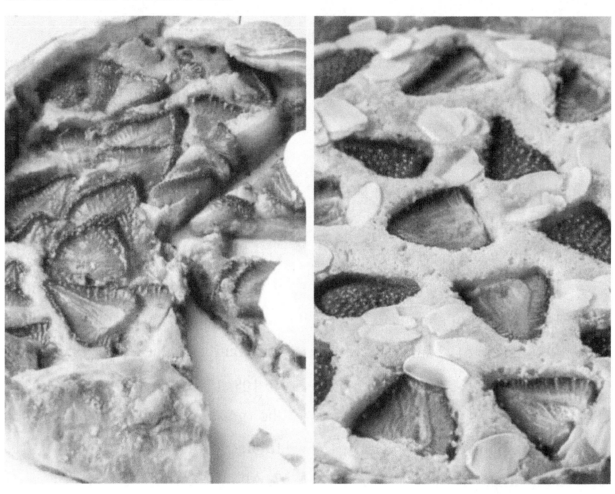

6. Pumpkin Oatmeal Cookies

These cookies are a nutritious snack that contains pumpkin, which is high in fiber and beta-carotene, as well as oats, which are good for heart health.

INGREDIENTS:

- 2 cups all-purpose flour
- 1 1/3 cups oats
- 1 teaspoon baking soda
- 1 teaspoon cinnamon
- 1/2 teaspoon salt
- 1 cup butter, softened
- 1 cup sugar
- 1 cup brown sugar
- 1 cup canned pumpkin
- 1 teaspoon vanilla extract
- 3/4 cup chopped walnuts
- 3/4 cup raisins
- 1 egg

INSTRUCTIONS:

1. Heat the oven to 350°F.

2. Combine the flour, oatmeal, baking soda, cinnamon, and salt.

3. Cream together the butter and sugars; then add the egg, pumpkin, and vanilla.

4. Gradually add the dry ingredients, stirring in the walnuts and raisins.

5. Place dough on a baking sheet and bake for 14-16 minutes.

COOKING TIPS:

1. To make chewier biscuits, remove as much moisture from the pumpkin puree as possible.

2. To make thicker cookies, refrigerate the dough for 30 minutes before baking

Nutritional Values Per Serving: Calories: 120 | Fat: 5g | Carbohydrates: 16g | Protein: 2g | Fiber: 1g

SERVING PORTION: MAKES ABOUT 24 COOKIES.

PREP TIME: 15 MINUTES.

COOK TIME: 16 MINUTES.

7. Cherry Almond Scones

A prostate cancer diet for seniors should contain foods high in antioxidants, fiber, and healthy fats. These scones contain almonds, which are rich in healthy fats and vitamin E, an antioxidant.

INGREDIENTS:

- 2 cups of self-raising flour
- 1/4 cup of caster sugar
- 1/2 cup of cold butter, cubed
- 3/4 cup of buttermilk
- 1/2 cup of dried cherries
- 1/4 cup of sliced almonds
- 1 tsp. of almond extract
- Milk for glazing
- Flaked almonds and demerara sugar for topping (optional)

INSTRUCTIONS:

1. Heat the oven to 220°C (425°F).

2. Sift flour into a mixing bowl, then add sugar.

3. Rub in the butter until it resembles breadcrumbs.

4. Combine the buttermilk, cherries, and almond essence, stirring to make a soft dough.

5. Turn out onto a floured surface, knead lightly, and shape into a circular approximately 2 cm thick.

6. Using a cutter, cut into scones, lay on a baking tray, brush with milk, and sprinkle with almonds and sugar if desired.

7. Bake for 12 to 15 minutes, or until risen and golden.

COOKING TIPS:

1. Keep all ingredients as cold as possible to get a flaky scone.

2. Avoid overworking the dough to keep the scones light.

Nutritional Values Per Serving: Calories: 200 | Fat: 9g | Carbohydrates: 26g | Protein: 4g | Fiber: 1g

SERVING PORTION: MAKES ABOUT 8 SCONES.

PREP TIME: 15 MINUTES. COOK TIME: 15 MINUTES.

8. Berry Bread Pudding

This dessert contains berries, which are strong in antioxidants and may help fight oxidative stress, which is good for prostate health.

INGREDIENTS:

- 8 cups of cubed day-old bread
- 2 cups of mixed berries (strawberries, raspberries, and blueberries)
- 4 large eggs
- 3/4 cup of sugar
- 2 cups of half-and-half
- 1 tsp. of vanilla extract
- 1/2 tsp. of almond extract

INSTRUCTIONS:

1. Heat the oven to 175°C (350°F).

2. Butter a baking dish and sprinkle it with sugar.

3. Mix the eggs, sugar, and a bit of salt until smooth.

4. Stir in the half-and-half and extracts, then add the bread cubes.

5. Let it soak for 15 minutes before pouring it into the baking dish.

6. Top with berries and bake for approximately an hour, or until set.

COOKING TIPS:

1. For a more flavorful bread, use brioche or challah.

2. Allow the bread to soak completely for a creamier texture.

Nutritional Values Per Serving: Calories: 250 | Fat: 10g | Carbohydrates: 35g | Protein: 6g | Fiber: 2g

SERVING PORTION: SERVES 8.

PREP TIME: 20 MINUTES (PLUS 15 MINUTES SOAKING TIME).

COOK TIME: 1 HOUR.

9. Baked Potato Crisps

Potatoes are rich in vitamins and fiber. Baking them rather than frying lowers the cholesterol level, making it a better option for a prostate cancer diet.

INGREDIENTS:

- 2 large russet potatoes
- 1 tablespoon of olive oil
- 1/2 teaspoon of sea salt
- Optional: black pepper, paprika, or dried herbs for seasoning

INSTRUCTIONS:

1. Heat the oven to 425°F (220°C).

2. Cut the potatoes into thin slices using a mandoline or sharp knife.

3. Toss the slices with olive oil and salt, then place them on a baking sheet.

4. Bake for 15-20 minutes, until crispy and golden brown.

5. Allow it to cool and crisp up more.

COOKING TIPS:

1. Soak potato slices in water for 30 minutes before baking to remove excess starch and increase crispiness.

2. To ensure equal cooking, do not overlap the slices on the baking pan.

Nutritional Values Per Serving: Calories: 150 | Fat: 3.5g | Carbohydrates: 26g | Protein: 3g | Fiber: 2g

SERVING PORTION: SERVES 4.

PREP TIME: 10 MINUTES (PLUS SOAKING TIME).

COOK TIME: 20 MINUTES.

10. Crunchy Sunflower Seed Granola

Sunflower seeds are high in antioxidants and vitamin E, making them a great option for a prostate-friendly diet. This granola is also high in fiber and contains healthy fats.

INGREDIENTS:

- 3 cups of rolled oats
- 1 cup of sunflower seeds
- 1/2 cup of honey or maple syrup
- 1/4 cup of coconut oil
- 1 teaspoon of vanilla extract
- 1/2 teaspoon of cinnamon
- Pinch of salt

INSTRUCTIONS:

1. Preheat the oven to 300°F (150° C).

2. In a big bowl, combine all of the ingredients thoroughly.

3. Transfer the mixture to a baking sheet and bake for 30-40 minutes, stirring regularly.

4. Allow it to cool fully to harden.

COOKING TIPS:

1. After baking, add dried fruit or nuts for extra flavor and nutrition.

2. Keep in an airtight container to retain crunchiness.

Nutritional Values Per Serving: Calories: 210 | Fat: 10g | Carbohydrates: 26g | Protein: 6g | Fiber: 4g

SERVING PORTION: SERVES 6.

PREP TIME: 10 MINUTES.

COOK TIME: 40 MINUTES.

11. Butternut Squash Bites

Butternut squash has high levels of vitamins A and C, as well as fiber and potassium. These nibbles are a delicious way to get the benefits of squash in a prostate-friendly diet.

INGREDIENTS:

- 1 butternut squash, peeled and cubed
- 2 tablespoons of olive oil
- 1 teaspoon of sage, chopped
- Salt and pepper to taste
- 1/4 cup of grated Parmesan cheese
- 1/4 cup of breadcrumbs
- Optional: pumpkin seeds for garnish

INSTRUCTIONS:

1. Heat the oven to 375°F (190°C).

2. Mix the butternut squash cubes with olive oil, sage, salt, and pepper.

3. Combine the Parmesan cheese and bread crumbs, then coat the squash cubes with the mixture.

4. Place on a baking pan and bake for 25–30 minutes or until brown and soft.

5. Optionally, garnish with pumpkin seeds before serving.

COOKING TIPS:

1. For added crispiness, broil the bits for the last 2-3 minutes.

2. Space the squash cubes apart on the baking pan to ensure uniform roasting.

Nutritional Values Per Serving: Calories: 90 | Fat: 4g | Carbohydrates: 12g | Protein: 2g | Fiber: 2g

SERVING PORTION: MAKES ABOUT 24 BITES.

PREP TIME: 15 MINUTES.   COOK TIME: 30 MINUTES.

12. Guacamole with Whole Grain Tortilla Chips

Avocados are high in healthy fats and fiber, making them ideal for a heart-healthy diet. This snack served with whole-grain tortilla chips, is both enjoyable and nutritious.

INGREDIENTS:

- 3 ripe avocados
- Juice of 1 lime
- 1/4 cup of red onion, finely chopped
- 1/4 cup of fresh cilantro, chopped
- 1 jalapeño, seeded and minced
- Salt to taste
- Whole grain tortilla chips

INSTRUCTIONS:

1. Half the avocados and remove the pits. Scoop the meat into a basin.

2. Combine lime juice, red onion, cilantro, jalapeños, and salt.

3. Using a fork, mash the ingredients together while leaving some lumps for texture.

4. Serve immediately with whole-grain tortilla chips.

COOKING TIPS:

1. To preserve the guacamole green, place plastic wrap instantly on the surface before serving.

2. Add chopped tomatoes for a pop of color and other nutrition.

Nutritional Values Per Serving: Calories: 150 | Fat: 12g | Carbohydrates: 10g | Protein: 2g | Fiber: 7g

SERVING PORTION: SERVES 4-6 AS AN APPETIZER.

PREP TIME: 10 MINUTES.

13. Trail Mix with Dried Fruits and Nuts

This trail mix is a nutritious, refreshing snack ideal for seniors. The dried fruits include fiber, vitamins, and antioxidants, while the nuts contain healthy fats and protein.

INGREDIENTS:

- 1 cup of dried fruits (like mango, strawberries, and blueberries)
- 1/2 cup of nuts (almonds or your favorite nuts)
- Optional: banana chips or seeds

INSTRUCTIONS:

1. In a large mixing bowl, add the dried fruits and nuts.

2. If desired, add banana chips or seeds to the mixture.

3. Keep in an airtight container or sealed bag for up to one month.

COOKING TIPS:

1. For the finest flavor and nutrients, use unsweetened and unsulfured dried fruits.

2. Toasting the nuts before adding them to the mixture might improve their taste.

Nutritional Values Per Serving: Calories: 200 | Fat: 10g | Carbohydrates: 30g | Protein: 5g | Fiber: 4g

SERVING PORTION: MAKES ABOUT 10 SERVINGS.

PREP TIME: 5 MINUTES.

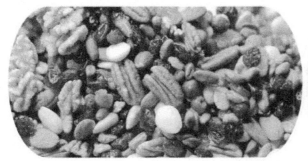 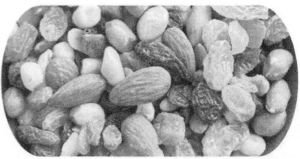

14. Roasted Chickpeas with Spices

Roasted chickpeas are a crispy and delicious snack that is high in protein and fiber. They're a great alternative to processed food and may be seasoned in a variety of ways to suit your tastes.

INGREDIENTS:

- 2 cans (15-ounce each) of chickpeas, drained and dried
- 2 tablespoons of olive oil
- 1/2 teaspoon each of cumin, chili powder, and salt

INSTRUCTIONS:

1. Heat the oven to 400°F (200°C).

2. Toss the chickpeas with olive oil and seasonings until well coated.

3. Arrange on a baking sheet in a single layer.

4. Roast for 20–35 minutes, or until crispy and golden brown.

COOKING TIPS:

1. To ensure crispiness, make sure the chickpeas are very dry before roasting.

2. To add variation, use other spices such as paprika, garlic powder, or curry powder.

Nutritional Values Per Serving: Calories: 150 | Fat: 6g | Carbohydrates: 20g | Protein: 6g | Fiber: 5g

SERVING PORTION: SERVES 4.

PREP TIME: 10 MINUTES.   COOK TIME: 35 MINUTES.

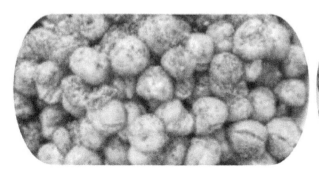
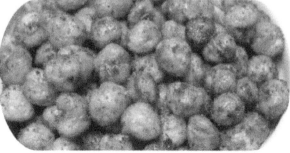

15. Pop Sorghum Trail Mix

Popsorghum is a light and airy snack that's a great alternative to popcorn. It's gluten-free and goes great with a variety of toppings for a filling trail mix.

INGREDIENTS:

- 1/2 cup of popped sorghum
- 1/4 cup of coconut shreds
- 1/4 cup of dark chocolate chips
- 3 tablespoons of hemp seeds
- 1/4 cup walnuts

INSTRUCTIONS:

1. Microwave the sorghum in a brown paper bag for 2–3 minutes.

2. Combine popped sorghum with coconut shreds, chocolate chips, hemp seeds, and walnuts.

3. Place in an airtight container or ziploc bag.

PREP TIPS:

1. You can use any nuts or seeds you choose in this recipe.

2. Include dried fruit for added sweetness and fiber.

Nutritional Values Per Serving: Calories: 200 | Fat: 12g | Carbohydrates: 18g | Protein: 5g | Fiber: 3g

SERVING PORTION: SERVES 4.

PREP TIME: 10 MINUTES.

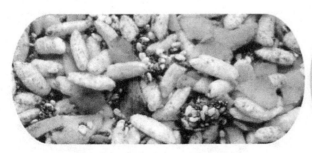 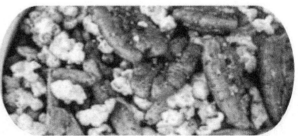

CHAPTER 7: PROSTATE FRIENDLY SMOOTHIE DIET

1. Chocolate Hazelnut Smoothie

This smoothie mixes the rich flavors of chocolate and hazelnuts. Hazelnuts include a variety of beneficial fats, vitamins, and minerals, including vitamin E, an antioxidant. The cocoa imparts a soothing chocolate taste while also providing antioxidants.

INGREDIENTS:

- 1 cup of almond milk
- 1/4 cup of rolled oats
- 2 tablespoons of chocolate-hazelnut spread
- 1 teaspoon of espresso powder (optional)
- 1 ripe banana
- 1/2 cup of ice cubes

INSTRUCTIONS:

1. Mix the almond milk, oats, chocolate-hazelnut spread, espresso powder (if using), banana, and ice in a blender.

2. Blend on high until completely smooth.

3. Pour into a glass and serve immediately.

PREP TIPS:

1. To get a smoother texture, soak the oats in the almond milk for 15-30 minutes before blending.

2. If you want a less sweet smoothie, reduce the amount of chocolate hazelnut spread.

Nutritional Values Per Serving: Calories: Approximately 350-400 | Fat: 17g | Carbohydrates: 50g | Protein: 8g | Fiber: 6g

SERVING PORTION: SERVES 1-2.

PREP TIME: 5 MINUTES.

2. Banana and Peanut Butter Protein Smoothie

This smoothie has plenty of protein and healthy fats, making it a good choice for seniors on a prostate cancer diet. Bananas provide potassium and fiber, while peanut butter contains protein and heart-healthy monounsaturated fats.

INGREDIENTS:

- 2 ripe bananas
- 2 tablespoons of peanut butter
- 1 cup of almond milk
- Optional: 1 tablespoon flaxseed or chia seeds for added fiber

INSTRUCTIONS:

1. Place bananas, peanut butter, and almond milk in a blender.
2. Blend until smooth.
3. For added fiber, blend in flaxseed or chia seeds until well combined.

COOKING TIPS:

1. Use frozen bananas for a thicker, creamier texture.
2. If you prefer a sweeter taste, add a touch of honey or maple syrup.

Nutritional Values Per Serving: Calories: 325 | Fat: 16g | Carbohydrates: 40g | Protein: 8g | Fiber: 5g

SERVING PORTION: SERVES 2.

PREP TIME: 5 MINUTES.

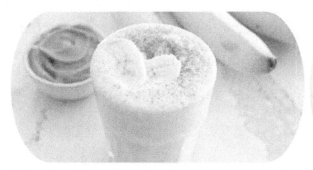
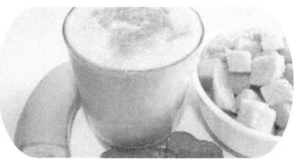

3. Spinach and Pineapple Detox Smoothie

This detox smoothie has antioxidants and vitamins from spinach and pineapple. It's an enjoyable and clean drink that is also hydrating and good for your prostate.

INGREDIENTS:

- 1 cup of fresh spinach
- 1 cup of frozen pineapple chunks
- 1 banana
- 1 cup of water or coconut water

INSTRUCTIONS:

1. Add spinach and liquid to the blender and blend until smooth.

2. Add pineapple and banana, and blend again until creamy.

PREP TIPS:

1. Add ice to make your smoothie cooler and more refreshing.

2. Adjust the amount of liquid to get the required consistency.

Nutritional Values Per Serving: Calories: 180 | Fat: 1g | Carbohydrates: 45g | Protein: 2g | Fiber: 4g

SERVING PORTION: SERVES 2.

PREP TIME: 5 MINUTES.

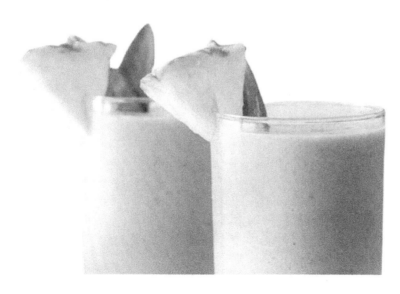

4. Cranberry Smoothie

Cranberries are recognized for numerous health benefits, including urinary tract health, which can be especially useful for prostate health. This smoothie balances the sharpness of cranberries with the sweetness of other fruits.

INGREDIENTS:

- 1/2 cup of fresh cranberries
- 1/2 cup of frozen mixed berries
- 1 banana
- 1 cup almond milk

INSTRUCTIONS:

1. Mix all the ingredients in a blender.
2. Blend until smooth and creamy.

PREP TIPS:

1. If the smoothie is too tart, sweeten it with a small amount of honey or maple syrup.
2. To make the smoothie thicker, add a frozen banana.

Nutritional Values Per Serving: Calories: 160 | Fat: 2g | Carbohydrates: 35g | Protein: 2g | Fiber: 5g

SERVING PORTION: SERVES 2.

PREP TIME: 5 MINUTES.

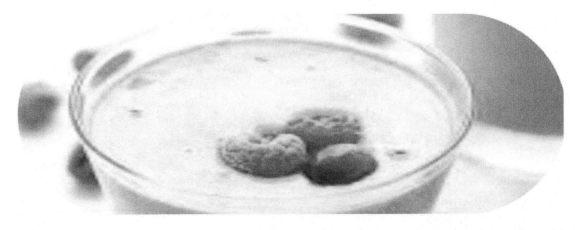

5. Carrot Cake Smoothie

This smoothie is high in beta-carotene from carrots, which is beneficial to eye health and contains antioxidants. It's a delicious dessert that tastes similar to carrot cake but without the extra sugar.

INGREDIENTS:

- 1 large, ripe frozen banana
- 1 small carrot, chopped
- 1/4 tsp. of ground cinnamon
- 1/2 tsp. of vanilla extract
- 1 tsp. of fresh minced or grated ginger
- A pinch of ground nutmeg
- 1/2 - 1 cup of dairy-free milk (adjust for desired thickness)
- Optional: 1 pitted date for extra sweetness

INSTRUCTIONS:

1. Combine all the ingredients in a high-speed blender.
2. Blend until creamy and smooth.
3. Adjust the amount of dairy-free milk to your desired consistency.

PREP TIPS:

1. Freeze the carrot as well to create a thicker, colder smoothie.
2. If you don't have a date, add some honey or maple syrup to sweeten it.

Nutritional Values Per Serving: Calories: 250 | Fat: 1g | Carbohydrates: 60g | Protein: 3g | Fiber: 6g

SERVING PORTION: SERVES 1.

PREP TIME: 5 MINUTES.

6. Watermelon and Mint Smoothie

Watermelon is hydrating, while mint has digestive benefits. This smoothie is ideal for hot days and makes a nice, light snack.

INGREDIENTS:

- 2 cups of cubed watermelon, frozen
- 1/4 cup of fresh mint leaves
- Juice of 1 lime
- 1 tbsp. of honey (optional)

INSTRUCTIONS:

1. Put all the ingredients in a blender.
2. Blend until smooth.
3. Serve immediately for the best flavor.

PREP TIPS:

1. To add extra coolness, add a couple of ice cubes to the mixer.
2. Adjust the honey to taste, based on the sweetness of the watermelon.

Nutritional Values Per Serving: Calories: 100 | Fat: 0g | Carbohydrates: 25g | Protein: 2g | Fiber: 1g

SERVING PORTION: SERVES 2.

PREP TIME: 5 MINUTES.

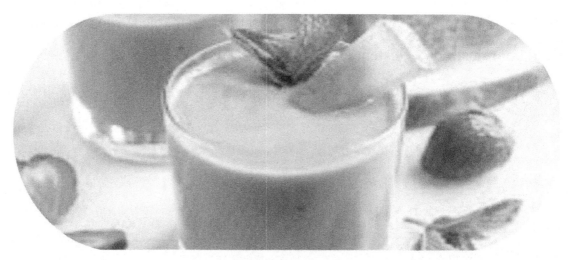

7. Pink Grapefruit Smoothie

Grapefruit is well-known for its high levels of vitamin C and lycopene, both of which are potent antioxidants. This smoothie is tart and delicious, with a lovely pink color.

INGREDIENTS:

- 1 pink grapefruit, peeled and seeded
- 1 sweet apple, cored and chopped
- 1 cup of strawberries, fresh or frozen
- A handful of fresh mint
- 8-10 ice cubes
- Optional: 1 teaspoon of date extract for sweetness

INSTRUCTIONS:

1. Mix all the ingredients in a blender.
2. Process until smooth.
3. Taste and add date extract if a sweeter smoothie is desired.

PREP TIPS:

1. If the smoothie is too thick, add a little water or almond milk to thin it up.
2. The mint may be changed to suit individual tastes.

Nutritional Values Per Serving: Calories: 180 | Fat: 1g | Carbohydrates: 45g | Protein: 2g | Fiber: 5g

SERVING PORTION: SERVES 2.

PREP TIME: 5 MINUTES.

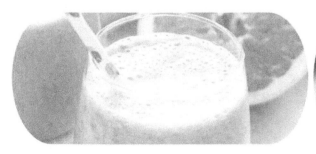
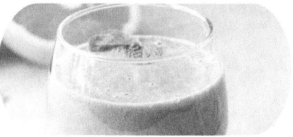

8. Pineapple Coconut Smoothie

This tropical smoothie has vitamin C and bromelain from pineapple, which may help with digestion and inflammation. Coconut has healthy cholesterol that promotes hormonal balance.

INGREDIENTS:

- 1 cup of frozen pineapple chunks
- 1 banana
- 1 cup of coconut milk
- Optional: Honey or maple syrup for sweetness

INSTRUCTIONS:

1. Put the pineapple, banana, and coconut milk in a blender.
2. Blend until smooth.
3. Taste and add honey or maple syrup, if desired.

PREP TIPS:

1. Use frozen pineapple to cool the smoothie without adding ice.
2. If the smoothie is too thick, add a little water or extra coconut milk to achieve the required consistency.

Nutritional Values Per Serving: Calories: 260 | Fat: 12g | Carbohydrates: 36g | Protein: 2g Fiber: 3g

SERVING PORTION: SERVES 2.

PREP TIME: 5 MINUTES.

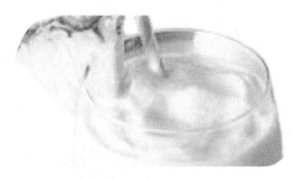
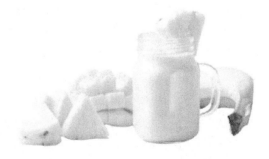

9. Blueberry and Almond Milk Smoothie

Blueberries are a superfood rich in antioxidants and phytonutrients. Almond milk is a dairy-free source of calcium and vitamin E, which are beneficial to skin and heart health.

INGREDIENTS:

- 1 1/2 cups of almond milk
- 1 1/2 cups of frozen blueberries
- 1 frozen banana
- 1/4 cup of almond butter
- 1/4 cup of old-fashioned oats

INSTRUCTIONS:

1. Mix all the ingredients in a blender.
2. Blend on high speed until smooth.
3. Serve immediately.

PREP TIPS:

1. Add the liquids first to aid in the mixing process.
2. If you want a sweeter smoothie, add a little honey or maple syrup.

Nutritional Values Per Serving: Calories: 300 | Fat: 15g | Carbohydrates: 40g | Protein: 8g | Fiber: 7g

SERVING PORTION: SERVES 2.

PREP TIME: 5 MINUTES.

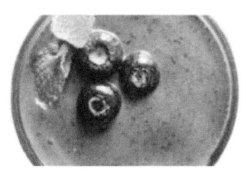 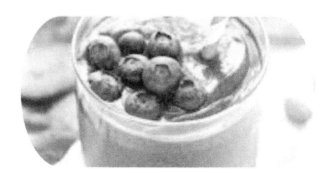

10. Kiwi and Orange Smoothie

Kiwi and orange form a vitamin C-rich smoothie that boosts the immune system. The natural sugars give a rapid energy boost, while the fiber supports digestion.

INGREDIENTS:

- 2 ripe kiwis
- Juice of 2 oranges
- 1 tablespoon of chia seeds
- 1/4 teaspoon of turmeric
- 1 teaspoon of honey
- 1 cup of water or coconut water
- 1/2 cup of ice

INSTRUCTIONS:

1. Peel the kiwis and cut them into quarters.
2. Squeeze the juice from the oranges.
3. Put all the ingredients in a blender.
4. Blend until smooth.

PREP TIPS:

1. Add the ice last to prevent over-blending and diluting the smoothie.
2. Adjust the sweetness with honey to your taste.

Nutritional Values Per Serving: Calories: 180 | Fat: 3g | Carbohydrates: 35g | Protein: 3g | Fiber: 5g

SERVING PORTION: SERVES 2.
PREP TIME: 5 MINUTES.

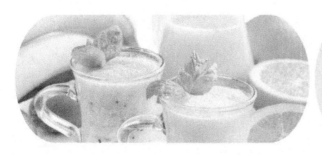
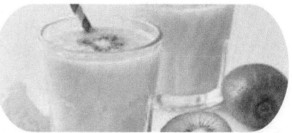

CHAPTER 8: 30-DAY PROSTATE CANCER RECOVERY MEAL PLAN

	BREAKFAST	LUNCH	DINNER	SNACKS
1	Quinoa Breakfast Bowl With Berries And Almond	Walnut Tomato Sauce with Zucchini Lasagna Noodles	Spaghetti Squash with Turkey Bolognese	Coconut and Date Energy Bites
2	Vegetable And Tofu Scramble	Shrimp Salad with Sun-Dried Tomato Vinaigrette	Ginger-Garlic Shrimp Stir Fry	Grilled Pineapple with Honey and Pistachios
3	Breakfast Burrito With Black Beans Salsa	Grilled Portbello Mushroom Salad	Grilled Vegetable and Chicken Kebabs	Dark Chocolate and Almond Clusters
4	Chia Seed Pudding With Mango	Lentil And Vegetable Soup	Zucchini Noodles with Pesto and Cherry Tomatoes	Baked Apples with Cinnamon and Walnuts
5	Oatmeal With Pecans And Dried Cranberries	Brown Rice Bowl With Teriyaki Salmon	Grilled Tofu and Vegetable Skewers	Strawberry-Almond Cream Tart
6	Almond Butter Banana Smoothie Bowl	Broccoli And Chedder Stuffed Baked Potatoes	Spinach and Mushroom Stuffed Chicken Breast	Pumpkin Oatmeal Cookies
7	Sweet Potato Hash With Turkey Sausage	Chickpea And Spinach Stew	Sweet and Spicy Grilled Shrimp	Cherry Almond Scones
8	Spinach And Feta Omellete	Barley and Vegetable Stir-Fry	Maple Glazed Ginger Brussels Sprouts	Berry Bread Pudding
9	Avocado Toast With Poached Egg	Quinoa Salad with Grilled Chicken	Vegetarian Enchilada Pasta	Baked Potato Crisps
10	Spinach And Mushroom Frittata	Quinoa and Black Bean Burrito Bowl	Turkey-Broccoli Stir-Fry	Crunchy Sunflower Seed Granola

	BREAKFAST	LUNCH	DINNER	SNACKS
11	Whole Grain Avocado Toast	Roasted Vegetable and Hummus Wrap	Sautéed Polenta with Butter Beans	Butternut Squash Bites
12	Sautéed Chard with Feta and Egg Breakfast Toast	Asian Pan Seared Salmon Salad	Parmesan Mushroom Casserole	Guacamole with Whole Grain Tortilla Chips
13	Southwest Vegetable Frittata	Pasta w/ Crispy Rosemary Chickpeas & Roasted Tomatoes	Balsamic Chicken With Pears	Trail Mix with Dried Fruits and Nuts
14	Strawberry Chia Smoothie	Herby Chicken Breasts	Thyme-Lemon Marinated Chicken	Roasted Chickpeas with Spices
15	Ricotta, Basil, Strawberry Toast	Salmon and Veggie Egg Muffins	Zucchini Noodles with Pesto and Cherry Tomatoes	Popsorghum Trail Mix
16	Vegetable And Tofu Scramble	Chickpea And Spinach Stew	Sautéed Polenta with Butter Beans	Coconut and Date Energy Bites
17	Quinoa Breakfast Bowl With Berries And Almond	Quinoa Salad with Grilled Chicken	Grilled Tofu and Vegetable Skewers	Grilled Pineapple with Honey and Pistachios
18	Chia Seed Pudding With Mango	Lentil And Vegetable Soup	Ginger-Garlic Shrimp Stir Fry	Baked Apples with Cinnamon and Walnuts
19	Oatmeal With Pecans And Dried Cranberries	Roasted Vegetable and Hummus Wrap	Spaghetti Squash with Turkey Bolognese	Dark Chocolate and Almond Clusters
20	Spinach And Feta Omellete	Brown Rice Bowl With Teriyaki Salmon	Maple Glazed Ginger Brussels Sprouts	Pumpkin Oatmeal Cookies

	BREAKFAST	LUNCH	DINNER	SNACKS
21	Whole Grain Avocado Toast	Barley and Vegetable Stir-Fry	Balsamic Chicken With Pears	Cherry Almond Scones
22	Breakfast Burrito With Black Beans Salsa	Asian Pan Seared Salmon Salad	Vegetarian Enchilada Pasta	Strawberry-Almond Cream Tart
23	Almond Butter Banana Smoothie Bowl	Pasta w/ Crispy Rosemary Chickpeas & Roasted Tomatoes	Thyme-Lemon Marinated Chicken	Baked Potato Crisps
24	Sweet Potato Hash With Turkey Sausage	Broccoli And Chedder Stuffed Baked Potatoes	Turkey-Broccoli Stir-Fry	Butternut Squash Bites
25	Avocado Toast With Poached Egg	Walnut Tomato Sauce with Zucchini Lasagna Noodles	Sweet and Spicy Grilled Shrimp	Guacamole with Whole Grain Tortilla Chips
26	Spinach And Mushroom Frittata	Shrimp Salad with Sun-Dried Tomato Vinaigrette	Grilled Vegetable and Chicken Kebabs	Crunchy Sunflower Seed Granola
27	Southwest Vegetable Frittata	Quinoa and Black Bean Burrito Bowl	Spinach and Mushroom Stuffed Chicken Breast	Berry Bread Pudding
28	Strawberry Chia Smoothie	Grilled Portbello Mushroom Salad	Parmesan Mushroom Casserole	Trail Mix with Dried Fruits and Nuts
29	Sautéed Chard with Feta and Egg Breakfast Toast	Herby Chicken Breasts	Zucchini Noodles with Pesto and Cherry Tomatoes	Roasted Chickpeas with Spices
30	Ricotta, Basil, Strawberry Toast	Salmon and Veggie Egg Muffins	Grilled Tofu and Vegetable Skewers	Popsorghum Trail Mix

Measurement Chart

VOLUME EQUIVALENTS (LIQUID)

US Standard	US Standard (Ounces)	Metric (Approximate)
2 tablespoons	1 fl. oz.	30 mL
¼ cup	2 fl. oz.	60 mL
½ cup	4 fl. oz.	120 mL
1 cup	8 fl. oz.	240 mL
1½ cups	12 fl. oz.	355 mL
2 cups or 1 pint	16 fl. oz.	475 mL
4 cups or 1 quart	32 fl. oz.	1 L
1 gallon	128 fl. oz.	4L

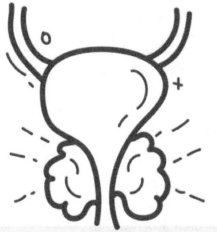

WEIGHT EQUIVALENTS

US Standard	Metric (Approximate)
½ ounce	15 g
1 ounce	30 g
2 ounces	60 g
4 ounces	115 g
8 ounces	225 g
12 ounces	340 g
16 ounces or 1 pound	455 g

OVEN TEMPERATURES

Fahrenheit (F)	Celsius (C) (Approximate)
250°F	120°C
300°F	150°C
325°F	165°C
350°F	180°C
375°F	190°C
400°F	200°C
425°F	220°C
450°F	230°C

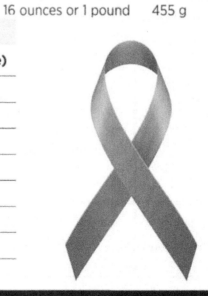

CHAPTER 9: PROSTATE CANCER EXERCISES FOR EASY RECOVERY IN SENIORS

- **Aerobic Exercise**

Walking:

1. Walking is a great low-impact aerobic activity for prostate cancer patients.

2. Aim for 90 minutes a week at a moderate pace.

3. Walking helps to strengthen your heart, enhance lung function, reduce tiredness, and control your weight.

4. Consider walking outside or on the treadmill.

- **Kegel Exercises**

Purpose: Kegel exercises focus on strengthening the pelvic floor muscles.

How to Perform Kegels:

1. Get comfortable or lie down.

2. Contract the muscles used to halt urinating (imagine stopping in midstream).

3. Hold the contraction for 5 seconds before releasing.

4. Repeat the cycle ten times, gradually increasing the length of each contraction.

Benefits: Kegels can enhance sexual function, urinary control, and overall pelvic health.

- **Stretching Exercises**

Purpose: Stretching maintains flexibility and prevents stiffness.

Recommended Stretches:

1. **Shoulder Stretches:** Reach one arm across your chest and gently pull it with the opposite hand.

2. **Triceps Stretches:** Extend one arm overhead and bend the elbow, reaching your hand down your back.

3. **Biceps Stretches:** Extend one arm straight in front of you and gently pull the fingers back.

Lower Back Stretches: Lie on your back, pull one knee toward your chest, and hold.

Perform these stretches daily to maintain joint and muscle flexibility.

- **Balance Exercises**

Purpose: Balance training helps counteract muscle imbalances and improve stability.

Key Balance Exercises:

1. **Standing on One Foot:** Stand on one leg for 30 seconds, then switch to the other leg. Use up 30 seconds each.

2. **Tightrope Walk:** Imagine walking on a tightrope, lifting your knees high for 5 seconds.

3. **Calf or Heel Raises:** Rise onto your toes (calf raises) or lift your heels (heel raises) for 30 seconds each.

4. **Grapevines:** Sidestep, crossing one foot behind the other.

Frequency: **Include balance exercises 2-3 times per week.**

- **Strength Training**

Purpose: Prevent muscle loss during cancer treatment.

Exercises:

1. **Bodyweight Squats:** Strengthen your legs by squatting down and standing up.

2. **Resistance Band Exercises:** Use bands for bicep curls, shoulder presses, and leg lifts.

3. **Light Dumbbell Exercises:** Perform seated or standing bicep curls, tricep extensions, and lateral raises.

Frequency: **Aim for 2-3 strength training sessions per week.**

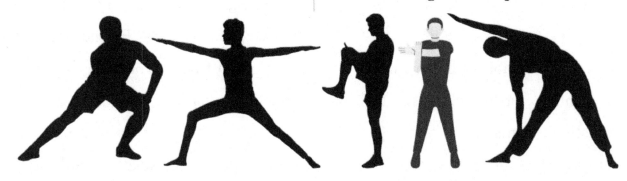

PROSTATE CANCER WORKOUT PLAN

DAY	STEPS TO FOLLOW
DAY 1	Cardio and Strength Cardio (15 minutes): Brisk Walking: Walk outdoors or on a treadmill for 15 minutes. Strength (6-minute routine): Abdominal Contractions: Tighten your abdominal muscles and hold for 3 breaths. Repeat 10 times. Wall Pushups: Stand facing a wall and do 10 pushups. Pelvic Tilts: Tilt your hips forward and backward. Repeat 8-12 times. Shoulder Blade Squeeze: Sit up straight and squeeze your shoulder blades together. Repeat 8-12 times. Toe Taps: Lift your toes while sitting in a chair. Repeat 20 times. Heel Raises: Keep your heels on the floor and lift your toes. Strengthen your calves.
DAY 2	Lower Body Strength and Balance Strength (Lower Body): Bodyweight Squats: 3 sets of 10 reps. Resistance Band Leg Lifts: Attach a resistance band to your ankle and lift your leg backward. 3 sets of 10 reps per leg. Balance: Standing on One Foot: Balance on one leg for 30 seconds. Switch legs. Tightrope Walk: Imagine walking on a tightrope, lifting your knees high. 3 sets of 10 steps. Calf Raises: Rise onto your toes. 3 sets of 10 reps.
DAY 3	Active Rest and Recovery Rest Day: Focus on gentle stretching and relaxation.

DAY 4	Upper Body and Core Strength Strength (Upper Body and Core): Bicep Curls: Use light dumbbells or resistance bands. 3 sets of 10 reps. Tricep Extensions: Extend your arms overhead and bend at the elbows. 3 sets of 10 reps. Seated Row: Sit on a chair and pull your arms back. 3 sets of 10 reps. Balance: Hip Opener: Stand on one leg and swing the other leg outward. 3 sets of 10 reps per leg.
DAY 5	Lower Body with Glute Emphasis Strength (Lower Body): Lunges: Forward or reverse lunges. 3 sets of 10 reps per leg. Glute Bridges: Lie on your back, lift your hips, and squeeze your glutes. 3 sets of 10 reps. Balance: Seated Row with Cross Punches: Sit on a chair and alternate punching forward. 3 sets of 10 reps.
DAY 6	Upper Body Strength Strength (Upper Body): Pushups: Wall pushups or modified pushups on your knees. 3 sets of 10 reps. Shoulder Press: Use light dumbbells or resistance bands. 3 sets of 10 reps.
DAY 7	Rest and Recovery Rest Day: Focus on gentle stretching and relaxation. **KINDLY RESHUFFLE THE WORKOUT BEST SUITABLE FOR YOU PROSTATE HEALTH**

CONCLUSION

"Prostate Cancer Cookbook for Seniors" is more than simply a collection of meals. It's a tapestry of food, empowerment, and hope woven together to help adults deal with the problems of prostate cancer.

As you turn each page, you are reminded of food's medicinal qualities. You're urged to adopt a new way of eating that's good for your health, respects your body, and helps you battle prostate cancer.

The recipes in this cookbook encourage you to taste the flavors, enjoy the textures, and appreciate the nutrition that each meal provides for your body and spirit. They highlight the beauty in simplicity, the delight in research, and the healing effects of well-picked and tenderly prepared foods.

As you embark on this gastronomic excitement, you will be reminded that you are not alone. You stand in solidarity with other seniors living with prostate cancer, as well as caregivers, loved ones, and healthcare providers. You all benefit from the collective wisdom of this cookbook, gaining strength from its pages, inspiration from its recipes, and comfort from its advice.

You find refuge in the kitchen. Cooking gives you a purpose. You will find healing in the foods you prepare. This book is more than just a compilation of recipes. It is a partner on your wellness path, providing nutrition for both the body and the soul.

May each food you cook be full of love, intention, and healing energy. May each mouthful serve as a reminder of your tenacity, persistence, and unshakable dedication to your health. Each moment spent in the kitchen serves as a reminder of food's ability to nourish, heal, and bring us together in a shared sense of hope and rebirth.

As you finish this recipe, take its teachings with you into your daily life. Continue to experiment with new flavors and ingredients, and embrace the healing effects of food as you face prostate cancer with grace, bravery, and a fresh sense of purpose.

We cook together. Together, we heal. Together, we flourish. Remember that you're not alone on this road. You are a member of a community that is cooking, healing, and growing together. Let us continue our adventure, one recipe at a time.

Notes:

_____

_____

_____

Observations:

_____

_____

Progress:

_____

_____

_____

_____

_____

_____

_____

Weekly Meal Plan

Date:	Workout:

Monday	Tuesday	Wednesday

Thursday	Friday	Saturday

Observation/Progressive Note :

Weekly Meal Plan

Date:	Workout:

Monday	Tuesday	Wednesday

Thursday	Friday	Saturday

Observation/Progressive Note :

Weekly Meal Plan

Date:

Workout:

Monday

Tuesday

Wednesday

Thursday

Friday

Saturday

Observation/Progressive Note :

Weekly Meal Plan

Date:	Workout:

Monday	Tuesday	Wednesday

Thursday	Friday	Saturday

Observation/Progressive Note :

Weekly Meal Plan

Date:	Workout:

Monday	Tuesday	Wednesday

Thursday	Friday	Saturday

Observation/Progressive Note :

Weekly Meal Plan

Date:	Workout:

Monday	Tuesday	Wednesday

Thursday	Friday	Saturday

Observation/Progressive Note :

Weekly Meal Plan

Date:	Workout:

Monday	Tuesday	Wednesday

Thursday	Friday	Saturday

Observation/Progressive Note :

Weekly Meal Plan

Date:	Workout:

Monday	Tuesday	Wednesday

Thursday	Friday	Saturday

Observation/Progressive Note :

Weekly Meal Plan

Date:	Workout:

Monday	Tuesday	Wednesday

Thursday	Friday	Saturday

Observation/Progressive Note :

Weekly Meal Plan

Date:	Workout:

Monday	Tuesday	Wednesday

Thursday	Friday	Saturday

Observation/Progressive Note :

Weekly Meal Plan

Date:

Workout:

Monday	Tuesday	Wednesday

Thursday	Friday	Saturday

Observation/Progressive Note :

Weekly Meal Plan

Date: Workout:

Monday

Tuesday

Wednesday

Thursday

Friday

Saturday

Observation/Progressive Note :

Weekly Meal Plan

Date:	Workout:

Monday

Tuesday

Wednesday

Thursday

Friday

Saturday

Observation/Progressive Note :

Weekly Meal Plan

Date:	Workout:

Monday	Tuesday	Wednesday

Thursday	Friday	Saturday

Observation/Progressive Note :

Weekly Meal Plan

Date:	Workout:

Monday	Tuesday	Wednesday

Thursday	Friday	Saturday

Observation/Progressive Note :

Weekly Meal Plan

Date:

Workout:

Monday	Tuesday	Wednesday

Thursday	Friday	Saturday

Observation/Progressive Note :

Weekly Meal Plan

Date:	Workout:

Monday	Tuesday	Wednesday

Thursday	Friday	Saturday

Observation/Progressive Note :

Weekly Meal Plan

Date:	Workout:

Monday	Tuesday	Wednesday

Thursday	Friday	Saturday

Observation/Progressive Note :

Weekly Meal Plan

Date:	Workout:

Monday	Tuesday	Wednesday

Thursday	Friday	Saturday

Observation/Progressive Note :

Weekly Meal Plan

Date:	Workout:

Monday	Tuesday	Wednesday

Thursday	Friday	Saturday

Observation/Progressive Note :

Made in the USA
Las Vegas, NV
21 November 2024

12199943R00090